Qualified To Do Anything
With Nothing

To Enid

G. W. Taylor

Gordon Taylor

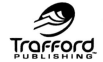

Trafford
PUBLISHING

Note for Librarians: A cataloguing record for this book is available from Library and Archives Canada at www. collectionscanada.ca/amicus/index-e.html
ISBN 1-4251-0373-1

Printed in Victoria, BC, Canada. Printed on paper with minimum 30% recycled fibre.
Trafford's print shop runs on "green energy" from solar, wind and other environmentally-friendly power sources.

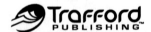

Offices in Canada, USA, Ireland and UK

Book sales for North America and international:
Trafford Publishing, 6E–2333 Government St.,
Victoria, BC V8T 4P4 CANADA
phone 250 383 6864 (toll-free 1 888 232 4444)
fax 250 383 6804; email to orders@trafford.com
Book sales in Europe:
Trafford Publishing (UK) Limited, 9 Park End Street, 2nd Floor
Oxford, UK OX1 1HH UNITED KINGDOM
phone +44 (0)1865 722 113 (local rate 0845 230 9601)
facsimile +44 (0)1865 722 868; info.uk@trafford.com
Order online at:
trafford.com/06-2130

10 9 8 7 6 5 4

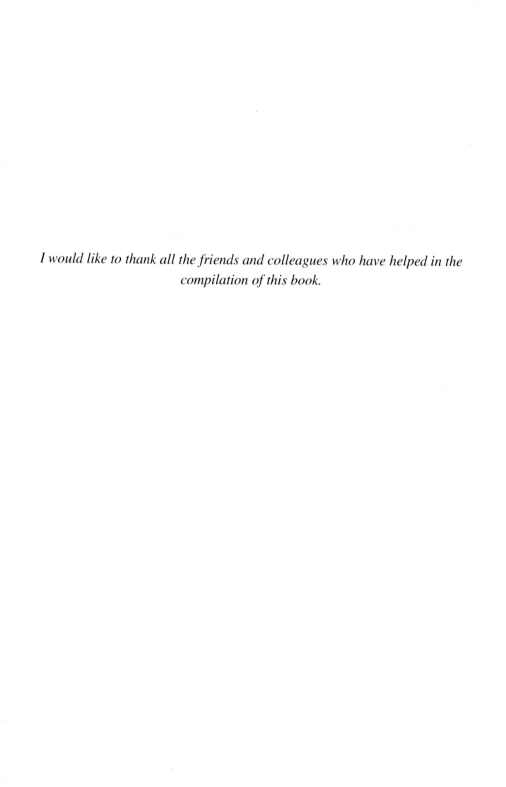

I would like to thank all the friends and colleagues who have helped in the compilation of this book.

Introduction

L et me say at the outset that I am a Residential Worker although at present I am in administration. I write from my own experience and that of colleagues in residential work. Since coming into this work I have read quite a number of books ostensibly dealing with residential work and on numerous occasions I have been amazed at some of the statements made in them and have often wondered how much practical experience the writer has had, as I know only too well that it bears no relation to the practicalities of this arduous and too often undervalued task. Residential work is unique insofar that it is a way of life rather than a job and since coming into the work realization has grown within me that there is a need for a book dealing with the practical side of this work.

I have thought about it for a long time, mainly because of the big problems of trying to put the intangibles, of which a great deal of this work is composed, into words. Since moving into administration and having to interview new staff and people of all ages wishing to make a career this work, I have realized that the need for a book of this type is still with us.

Only those of you who read the following pages will be able to judge whether or not my efforts have been worthwhile. If it opens the eyes of those who think that residential work is a soft option it will have been worth the effort.

All incidents are true, they have happened, are happening.

Prologue

R eading the newspapers and listening to the news it appears that juvenile crime is breaking all bounds and is becoming more and more vicious.

Care of the elderly seems to be very low down the list of priorities.

I spent many years of my life working and living in Approved Schools and later in management of both Homes for Children and Homes for the Elderly.

Working with children we were expected to "re-socialize" them! At that time all sanctions were being withdrawn. this was the start of the present day problems when we were forced to go down the long road which led to nowhere and cost many millions of pounds of public money. We are still travelling down the same road.

Whilst I was in the work local authorities were closing homes for the elderly as it was thought that this would save money and the same standard of care could be administered to the elderly in their own homes. This has proved not to be the case and many old people are now finding life in their own homes to be almost impossible.

Most residential workers said that this was not the road to take and it has since been proved that it is far more expensive and far less effective than taking the elderly into care.

The manuscript of this book was written almost twenty-five years ago but I was warned off getting it published as it was said I would never work again.

The book is about residential social work in which I was employed and tries to highlight the misleading books published at the time and show that the practicalities of the work bore no resemblance to what the books said. It was, and probably still is, a contentious book as it highlights the ignorance of people who sought to influence the ways in which different cases were handled but had no real knowledge of the effects upon the individual persons. These writers were regarded as the gurus of residential social services but in the main were preaching theory and not practice.

I set out to discredit those who were not honest enough to write the whole truth and who influenced Government thinking.

After being warned off publishing I used the manuscript for training purposes.

We the willing, led by the unknowing were doing the impossible for the ungrateful. We did so much with so little for so long that we are now qualified to do anything with nothing.

Chapter 1

When you come into residential work you take on the world. You will need the wisdom of Solomon, the stamina of an athlete and the patience of Job. It is a public centred occupation and in your everyday dealings with residents be they children, old people, mentally handicapped or whatever, you walk a razor's edge through a maze, a maze created by some faceless person with little or no knowledge at all of what it is like to live twenty four hours a day with anything from nine to a hundred anti-social, disturbed, deprived children or incontinent, confused, disabled elderly.

The only guidelines you have are, Thou shalt not kick, kiss or cuddle. This may not make sense to you but be patient and read on, hopefully it will become clearer. Field social workers have a set of Laws and Acts of Parliament to work to and if they work within those they are reasonably safe. The residential worker has little or nothing to work on other than what I have said above and when I say children, I mean aged 0 to 18 years when they usually go out of care. As I have said, you walk a razor's edge and this is no exaggeration. If you fall one way the media will tear you to pieces and if you fall the other way your Authority will be down on you, having put their own umbrella up first. You are condemned before you have a chance to speak; in fact you are guilty until you prove yourself innocent for you will find very few who will help. I admit we are not the only occupation where this kind of situation prevails but as far as I know it is the only one where you live with it twenty four hours a day. Others can finish their time and go home, hopefully to unwind.

One piece of advice I always give to anyone coming into residential work is get yourself a house, flat or caravan, anything to get you away from the premises but have a bolt hole somewhere. If you don't you will soon begin to wonder why you are becoming aggressive and short tempered. The strain of coping with a group of difficult children has to be experienced to be believed and while you live on the premises even when you are off duty you will be working, because as soon as you show yourself some child with whom you have a relationship will want you and you will be a very hard person if you chase them away with "I'm off duty, go and see so and so". I worked with one man who had considerable experience in this work who told me what I am telling you and I have found that it pays. He used to hitch up his caravan and drive just nine miles down the road to a quiet site. In short get away and unwind or you will very soon find yourself mentally and physically drained.[1:74]

When you enter residential work you may do so with "fire in your belly" and a feeling that you are going to change the world. Let me tell you now that you won't because the system will not let you. Don't ask me to describe what the system is, because it is a conglomerate of so many things, each one calculated to generate maximum frustration. What I can do is relate certain instances to you and hope you get the message.

I and my staff were taking a group of children, 11 to 14, away on holiday to the seaside. The children had all been committed by the courts. Now if you take children to the seaside they naturally expect to go swimming and prior to the holiday were full of what they were going to do. However, I was called to the office the week before we left and the conversation went something like this:

"Ah Mr Taylor you are taking some children on holiday next week".

"That's right".

"Where are you going?"

"Blank on sea".

"I presume you will be going swimming?"

"Yes, hopefully".

"I suppose you know what the rules are about this?"

"I don't follow you".

"Let me explain. (a rather fat file was produced). It states here that if a child in the care of a local authority is taken swimming in the sea, certain precautions must be taken. (reasonable). The person in charge must have a whistle (again reasonable) and children must wear a lifebelt and be attached to a responsible member of staff by a length of line and must not be allowed to go out more than fifty yards".

Imagine that with fifteen children and two male staff. I am not counting female staff who came.

Needless to say I put my head on the block and we went swimming our way, some of the children didn't wait to put on a swimming costume but just ran in fully clothed!

If I wanted to take children to the swimming baths either my wife or another member of staff would have to come as well. One would patrol round the sides in order that the other could play with the children. This in spite of what all the books say about good child care practice and forming meaningful relationships.

I was once accused by a Home Office Inspector of only giving the children a minority choice. He did not say it to me but to my Headmaster. At the time the ratio of boys to staff was 5 to 1 and I had fifteen boys on my own. He did not say, of course, that had anything happened to any of the boys or if any of them were in mischief I would have been on the carpet and asked to explain what I had been doing. Like so many others in similar positions he was prepared to make valued judgement on a few hours acquaintance and on a group of boys I had only known for a few months. Eventually they did go out alone within the school campus, played football and cricket unsupervised and tended their gardens. He should have returned twelve months later he might have learned something. This kind of event is not unusual from people who have attained the dizzy heights of officialdom, perhaps it is the rarefied atmosphere. Residential staff will talk honestly between themselves about their attitudes and feelings for the work but when anyone who smacks of officialdom arrives they will make the 'noises' the official wants to hear and he will go away feeling quite smug that the edicts handed down from the ivory towers are bearing fruit. Little does he known that these edicts were 'filed' in the wastepaper basket. Don't get the wrong idea. Residential workers are always looking for ways to help them to do their job better, but get disgusted when people with no real experience in the work start telling them how it should be done. This feeling extends to students and tutors but more of that later.[2]

One approved school I worked in had its own swimming bath. I was taking some boys for a swim one afternoon. While they were getting undressed I remarked on the absence of swimming trunks. I was told by the boys that they did not have any. I told them to get dressed as there would be no swimming in the nude. I went to the Matron (wife of the headmaster) and asked about the trunks. She seemed surprised that anyone should bother about such things but I got them eventually when she had knocked the dust off them. The boys told me later that they had never used the trunks before and always swam naked. Not only that but the Matron was in the habit of swimming at the same time-she of course always wore a costume. I took this statement with the proverbial grain of salt until it was later verified by a member of staff who had been there a number of years. None of the boys in this school was under sixteen.

There was a boy there who related to none of the staff. He was passionately fond of animals and birds and always had one or the other somewhere. Shortly after I had started at the school the boy found out that I had been an instructor in outdoor pursuits. Through this I formed quite a strong relationship with this particular boy as he took every opportunity to talk to me about climbing and canoeing. I was able to persuade him to let his 'pets' go free. I just asked him how he liked being where he was, well knowing what his answer would be and I pointed out to him that while he longed for the wild lonely places they belonged there and that he should allow them to live free. He was a boy of tremendous spirit and I was aware of the limits of our relationship. One day when I went on duty he was like a snarling beast and would allow no one near him and I could see from his face that he had been crying. I spoke to the other boys and discovered what the trouble was. I was told that he had found a young magpie which had fallen from the nest and not knowing which nest it was from he had decided to look after it until it was big enough to fend for itself. Of course it needed feeding frequently and while in class he had asked if he could go and feed the bird. The request was denied. This happened three times and the boy walked from the class and fed the bird. When he returned the teacher rounded on him and raved and ranted about his 'pets' (he only had one). In a raging temper the teacher went out and killed the young bird. This boy was seventeen and had a deep distrust of people and that teacher certainly did not help. I managed to repair my relationship with him so much so that one Christmas our Headmaster sent a member of staff to my house. I had left the school by this time but lived close by. I was asked if my wife and I would have the boy over the holiday as they wanted to close the school and the boy refused to go home. A lot of people tried to break the boy's spirit but the trouble was they couldn't tell the difference between spirit and delinquency.

The Headmaster suffered from what I call the 'New Society Syndrome'. Each time a new idea was written about in New Society he must try it. In fairness to him he was not the only one and there are still a lot like him. There were so many insufficiently considered projects under way they were doomed to failure even if they had gone on long enough which they did not. I knew I had got a post there because of my experience in outdoor activities but the significance of this did not strike me for a while. Intermediate Treatment was hitting the headlines at the time and it was put to me that I could make use of my talents. I said I would be happy to and told him what I would need in the way of equipment. He nearly had a fit, he fondly imagined that you just went in what you stood up in and all you needed for climbing was a clothes line. However, I formed an outdoor group and the boy I mentioned earlier was the first to join. Unfortunately as he was always in trouble he was on restrictions when I took a group away from school for a weekend. They all thought they were real tough guys but after carrying a heavy rucksack for a few hours in the mountains they began to cry enough. In spite of this the weekend was a huge success and word soon got around. I told the boy he would have to get off restrictions before he could come. It did not take him long and he came the second time out. One of my group got into trouble in school and a senior member of staff said to me. "Your Intermediate Treatment hasn't done much good has it?" We had only been out twice! I had about thirty boys in the group not all from my unit and all the time the group functioned not one of the thirty absconded. That was never mentioned. It was not long before I realised that I had been taken in about this activity. I worked two weekends out of three and I found that it was on my weekend off that I was expected to take a group out. This meant that my wife and son rarely went out anywhere. I had a long talk with the boys about it and they proved to be very understanding and we did not go out as often but we did go. The Headmaster would not agree to my taking a group out while I was on duty unless I took all thirty. The fact that the accepted safe number for one person to lead was ten made no difference to him nor did the fact that we had only three three man tents.

There was a young boy about twelve years old. We will call him Carl. His mother was dead and his father was cohabiting with a woman who had borne him four further children. In two years the boy had not had a letter from home. He went home on leave at regular intervals and usually failed to return. He did not stay at home but absconded and it was quite surprising how far he got. At that time it was usual for parents to sign and return a printed slip accepting responsibility for their child whilst they were at home. Every Monday without fail Carl would write a letter and send the form and every Saturday he would put on his good clothes and wait for the post to arrive and each Saturday he was disappointed. He would wait until 11 or 12 o'clock and then go and change. Sometimes he would weep when he thought he was alone for he was usually the only child left. To get him home for holidays the form had to be sent to the Field Worker who would take it to be signed and return it. Once when Carl failed to return a member of staff went through the usual procedure of going to his home first to see if he was there. The staff member knocked at the door which was opened by a little girl of about four or five wearing only a ragged slip. She was asked if her mum and dad were in but said they were out. The staff member went in to see if Carl was there. The house was filthy and there were two other children, one about two was sleeping on an indescribably dirty mattress covered with old coats and there was a baby a few months old also filthy dirty. The little girl picked up a dirty feeding bottle and started to feed the baby. The staff member ascertained that Carl was not there. The Field Worker was contacted and the business reported to her. She went to see the father and co-habitee who said that they had only been gone a few minutes to try out a car they had acquired. She believed them and nothing more was done. At successive case reviews over a two year period the field worker was asked to arrange for a foster home for Carl as staff felt that a good home and some affection was what the boy needed. It was pointed out to her that the boy had never received a letter but she said that she had spoken to Carl's father about that and had been assured that letters were written regularly. The children's mail record was shown to her and Carl's page was blank. She said she would take it up. The next week all the children were excited when Carl actually got a letter of four lines. Fostering was resisted because the father and cohabitee told the field worker that they loved Carl and she, as always, believed them. Carl eventually went home and then on to a Senior Boys School. The last we heard of that boy was that he was in Borstal.*

Staff who had been involved with Carl still talk about him and the tears they shed for him each Saturday.

A boy of seventeen was returned to school by the police after absconding. The Housemaster on duty was a friend of mine and was sleeping in a room just outside the dormitory. About two o'clock he was awakened by what he thought was a fight. He ran into the dormitory to see the boy who had been returned running down between the beds and diving head first at the wall. He realised right away that it was the result of drugs. The boy had brought some in with him and had taken them. It took six strapping boys to hold him down, one on each arm and leg and two to sit on him. He was obviously in a bad way so the Housemaster buzzed the Matron and explained the problem. She duly arrived with a glass of water and an aspirin! Eventually a psychiatrist was contacted and he gave the boy an injection to neutralise the effects of the drug.

The following case is typical of problems that can be created for the residential worker by lack of co-operation. I shall call the boy Stan. He was brought into care and placed in a Family Group Home. After a time a case conference was called and his teacher from day school was invited. It was said by residential staff and teacher that more specialised care was needed and a residential school was suggested. The field worker was not happy about the

*   Borstal – a prison for young boys.

suggestion but agreed to apply for a place in a residential school. Teachers in day school found Stan to be so difficult they asked for advice in dealing with and helping him- they got neither. The residential staff admitted quite frankly that they had neither the facilities nor the expertise to deal with the boy. He would deliberately stand and urinate over the bed, on the floor, in someone's locker, in other people's shoes. He would play with his faeces; spread it over himself and on the walls. He would indulge in screaming fits and in blind temper he would bite, scratch and kick other children or staff. He would make unprovoked vicious attacks on anyone within range and often in temper would bang his head against the wall. Over a period of time staff of the home made a very slight improvement in his behaviour but this was not carried over into day school where he would urinate into a Wellington and then pour it over some unfortunate child's head. This, of course, meant that the school and home were continually trying to placate irate parents who demanded to know what was going to be done about Stan. At one case conference the psychologist suggested that staff and teachers should ignore him when he started but nothing was said about how staff should cope with seventeen other children who would see what they would interpret as "Stan getting away with it"[3]. The staff pointed out that due to this reaction from other children they were not prepared to go along with his suggestion. The staff of the home maintained that a one to one relationship was needed and even asked students in the home to try this but without much success mainly because the student could not cope with the situation and they were continually abused by Stan and frequently told to "F... Off" and yet the more attention he got the more he demanded. He would get up at 5a.m. and upset the other children by jumping on their beds and hitting them and staff were getting very weary of uproars first thing in the morning. He would hoard his own toys but break any others he could lay his hands on. One of his teachers was suspicious of his hearing ability and asked for a test. He was found to have an impairment in his hearing, his adenoids were removed and his hearing improved. He was sent for an E.E.G which showed some brain damage. The consultant described it as a form of epilepsy without fits. A teacher in Junior School felt she was getting somewhere with Stan and was rather flushed with her success. This was short lived as she could not cope with the demands he made on her and the relationship rapidly deteriorated. Another case conference was called and it was agreed that a close relationship was needed or a residential school. The psychiatrist agreed with the decision but the psychologist did not and so the pattern of Stan's behaviour continued with the staff at their wits end being told what to do by people who did not have to cope with the situation. After some months had elapsed another case conference was called only this time it was the Senior Social worker who disagreed.[4] This pattern went on for two years and when finally all were agreed that a residential school would be the answer it was found that Stan's name had never been put down for residential school. The most significant point is that the outcome of the boy's behaviour was predicted by the staff of the home when he was first admitted but was rejected by a field worker.[6]

Two small examples which illustrate the vulnerability of residential staff and the pressures the system places on them. John has a cold. Staff feel it is not too bad and send him to school. The teacher telephones the home and says, "John has a cold". The next day staff keep John off school to cover themselves. A housemother is doing some sewing and is being helped by one of the girls. They find they are running short of cotton. The housemother asks the child to go to the shop for a reel of cotton. Money is obtained from petty cash and the child instructed to get a receipt. Can you imagine how children feel when they have to obtain a receipt for something costing a few coppers? This sort of requirement on the part of authority makes absolute nonsense of all the child care teachings.

Two boys, brothers were taken into care and placed in a large Family Group Home. One I shall call Tom. The staff of the home were ordinary residential workers. The officer in charge and his wife had a great deal of experience but no formal qualifications as such. At the first case conference it was recommended and agreed that an assessment was required as it was thought that the boys were too maladjusted for a Family Group Home. They duly went to an Assessment Centre, quite a well known one where it is reported they completely disrupted the place and also broke into staff homes. The centre recommended that Tom, whom they considered to be the leader, should be placed in either an establishment which would exercise strict control or a school for the maladjusted. A place was found for him in a well known school for the maladjusted where he stayed for one term only. They returned him to the Family Group Home with the report that he was too maladjusted for them!! What they expected the staff at the Home to do heaven alone knows. He stayed in the Home for three months without attending school simply because the school would not take him. You try keeping your child off school for three months and see what happens.[7] Tom was then sent to another well known assessment centre who again recommended a Maladjustment placement. He was returned to the Home where he stayed for a few months more and again went to the Assessment Centre and from there was sent to a Junior Approved School but spent weekends and holidays in the Home. Now this would be a good point to bring in the residential staff's feelings about schools and special units closing for holidays etc. but that is something I want to develop later.

Let me quote some examples of apparent indifference on the part of administration which placed genuine residential workers in an untenable position and which to my mind is totally inexcusable.

A Home which had in care a family of mixed race children. When a West Indian woman applied for a post of housemother the Officer in charge and his wife were very pleased if only for the sake of this family. They soon found they had made a bad mistake. The woman soon showed she did not like children and least of all mixed race. Stories began to drift back to the officer in charge and wife about the children being beaten and cruelly treated whilst they were off the premises. These stories were reported to a Senior Officer in Administration but there was no investigation. There were rumours that a child had literally been thrown down the stairs and of children being beaten with a wet towel so no marks would show. This again was reported and again was ignored. The West Indian housemother began behaving in a peculiar fashion. She would bare her breasts and other parts of her body to the children at the same time telling them that she was different from them. The other staff noticed that she used the table cutlery less and less and instead she used her fingers. This went on until eventually she was taking handfuls of food and stuffing them into her mouth smearing her face in the process. It dawned on staff after a while that she was regressing. While we expect some children to regress to a certain degree grave problems are presented when a member of staff does it, particularly to such an extent. However this again was reported and ignored. In the end it was a Senior Housemother who managed to get the woman out. It happened by chance and if all the staff had not been at screaming pitch over the whole business it might never have happened. The West Indian woman was coming downstairs and made a remark about 'white honkys' which she did quite often. The Senior Housemother heard the remark and rounded on her making it quite plain that they were all fed up with her attitude. The Housemother started to cry "race" but was told in no uncertain manner that if "race" was or ever had been a problem she would not have got over the door in the first place. She left within a week and I will leave it to the psychologists to interpret her behaviour. If Senior Administrative Staff had not been so indifferent none of this need have happened.

A West Indian boy was admitted to a Senior Boys Approved School. It soon became apparent to staff that the boy 'had it made' for himself. He was deliberately obstructive and abusive to staff and also chose his time well, when he had an audience, preferably other boys. Whenever a member of staff took this boy to task he would draw attention to himself by shouting "Racist you are only saying this to me because I'm Black". The other boys soon made capital of this and discipline was in serious danger of breaking down. Complaints to Senior Staff and Administration brought forth the reply "Be careful what you say to him because we will be accused of being racist and that would be embarrassing". One day a member of staff was involved in an incident with the boy which brought forth the usual accusation. The member of staff being heartily fed up with the boy caught him by the shirt front and said "Look son, I don't give a damn what colour you are but it is people like you who get the negro a bad name in this country". The staff member was on the carpet and in defence of his action pointed out that if Senior Management had not been so cowardly he would not have been put in that position. He eventually gave in his notice. The boy? He went on to Borstal.

A seventeen year old delinquent girl was taken into care. She was from a problem family well known to the social services. The Senior Social Worker stated his intention of putting the girl into a small family group home. The Officer in charge of a big home who knew the girl well told the Senior that to put her where he intended would end in disaster as she would disrupt the home completely. The home in question was run by a woman who was dedicated to her children, in fact they were a credit to her and in short it was a happy settled home. The Senior ignored the advice and the girl was placed in the home and promptly absconded. When she failed to return and since it was getting late the Housemother being concerned for one of her charges went to try and find her calling al all the 'seedy dives' in the process. The girl came and went as she pleased and boasted to the other children about escapades. Every night for two weeks the housemother went around the town to find the girl. Eventually tired out and frustrated the Housemother went to see her Seniors including the Senior Social Worker and told them that she could not cope with the girl and that her behaviour was having an adverse effect on the other girls. She asked them to move the girl and was told it could not be done. The housemother said if the girl was not moved she would have to leave. She was told "Alright, you go". The housemother packed her bags and tearfully said goodbye to the other children. The very day after she had left the girl was taken from the Group Home and sent to her own home. This may seem like a small thing to some but look at it closely. To many residential workers and to me it was a tragedy that such a thing should be allowed to happen. Here you have a person who is devoted to her task and who was forced into the position where she had to abdicate and what about the children who had enjoyed a happy stable environment? Too often people in authority impose their will upon residential staff and in spite of what staff say will sacrifice the whole environment for the sake of one. So much for good child care practice! [8:10:11]

A young woman was employed as a Deputy in a Children's Home. After a week or two the Officer in charge met his Senior from the office and was asked how the Deputy was getting on. The Officer in charge said, "I have a suspicion she is paranoid but it is early days yet, I'll keep you posted". As the weeks went by it was found that the new Deputy had somewhat peculiar ideas about child care. Regular reports on her progress and attitudes were being sent to the office. On one occasion she allowed the children to take and eat the Sunday joint which had been cooked on the Saturday. The day after she refused to give the children any food which meant younger ones had to try and get some food from somewhere and they went begging from houses in the area. The Officer in Charge tried to reason with the young woman but got nowhere. He tried being nasty and he tried being nice but made no impression. A short while after the incident he met a man in residential care in the same authority who had in the past had this young woman working in his home and his comment was, "What are you doing having a lunatic like that working your place?" They had a discussion about the young woman and the officer in charge was very disturbed. Bear in mind all the time regular reports were being submitted to the office about the young woman's progress and although he knew he had a problem he had not realised how great the problem really was. The Officer in Charge went on holiday for two weeks leaving this woman in charge. There was also a student on placement who fortunately proved to be a sensible young man with his feet firmly on the ground. For the two weeks anarchy reigned and if it had not been for the student the children would have physically assaulted the young woman. When the officer in charge returned he contacted his senior and reported what had been happening whilst he had been away. The senior said "Fair enough, you did warn me. I'll get someone down to see you." The next day two people arrived in the Home and the officer in charge realised during the course of the discussion that he was being made out to be the ogre and the one in the wrong. This surprised him greatly in view of his regular reports. It was also made apparent that they wanted this young woman to stay. The Officer in Charge told them that he realised he did not have the authority to dismiss her but as Officer in Charge he did not think she was a suitable person to look after children. The two people from the office indicated that if the Officer in Charge were to take the matter further they would be very upset. He had no intention of taking the matter further and so the young woman stayed. A short time later a Housemother in charge of a Family Group Home left in some haste and with equal haste the young woman was moved into the vacant place. The Officer in Charge said to his senior, "Look! Watch her for she will need a lot of help". The senior said he would do that. The young woman only lasted a few months in this home. It was alleged that she could not handle money; she spent everything including the children's holiday money and had to be reimbursed.

The above case is indicative of the attitude of some administrators to residential work. It is a very difficult task to explain intangibles and all too often people in senior positions have little or no knowledge of what life is like in a residential home and those who have had the experience forget what they themselves went through. Any senior worth his or her salt should be able to put themselves in the position of staff and should not ask staff to do what they themselves cannot or will not do. I digress, this will form the basis for another chapter.

Some examples which serve to illustrate the frustration created for residential staff by people who have high qualifications and do not consider comments made by residential workers as being worthy of note.

A fifteen and a half year old girl with a young baby (three months) had an argument with the father concerned. Staff in the centre were notified that the girl had removed her baby from the nursery and that they could expect difficulties. The police were notified and the other children in the establishment were made secure. The Superintendent and the Housemother tried to physically restrain the girl who struck the Superintendent and broke her spectacles and then attacked the Housemother with a chair and burst blood vessels in her leg. At this time the police were in the building and moved to help. The girl gave a karate chop to the policeman who was trying to restrain her on the stairs; she then ran upstairs and jumped out of a second storey window, collected her baby from the bushes where she had hidden it. This was a November night and she had not thought of the physical problems of a baby on a cold night. Later when she was apprehended ten police were involved. By this time the G.P had been contacted and a psychiatrist was on standby. The G.P was not prepared to certify the girl even though he was in possession of information to the effect that the girl had smashed two previous establishments where she had been placed. The staff of the establishments said that they did not regard the girl's placements with them as appropriate. As is often the case they were ignored. However, the girl was taken to a remand situation and was kept in a secure room for two days. When released from the room she proceeded to create havoc in the centre. Residential staff had asked for a psychiatric oversight for this girl but the professional people brushed the idea aside.

A twelve year old very aggressive, highly disturbed girl who showed a distinct need for psychiatric oversight and was in care on a Place of Safety Order. Containment by relationship became an impossible task as the girl continued to show considerable physical aggression to other children, staff and property. On several occasions the Superintendent indicated to the psychiatric services the need for intensive oversight and medical assessment and on each occasion was simply told to "contain her". The occasion arose when the girl had to appear in Court and while in the court she attacked the Social worker and the Police. She was removed from the court and returned to the home. The staff of the home were expected to continue to care for the girl without any further assistance from the medical profession. After spending most of one day physically restraining this girl on the floor the Superintendent made a further request to the psychiatric unit for help. Without making any effort to go to the home to see the girl's behaviour for himself the psychiatrist asked for her to be taken to his surgery. After further restraints and calming influences this was done and at that eleventh hour the girl was considered suitable for admission to a Psychiatric Hospital.

A fourteen and a half year old boy brought before the Court was admitted into care for committing Grievous Bodily Harm. He had approached a couple and asked for a light for a cigarette. When this was refused he stabbed the young man and he had to be put into an intensive care unit. During the period he was on remand in the Observation and Assessment Centre he drew a knife on another boy and caused numerous fights and tried to attack staff.

At the preliminary discussion prior to a report for the Court, residential staff recommended six months detention centre which was the most severe sentence which could be given to a boy of this age. The psychologist and psychiatrist were against this and also against it was a residential student who because of the boy's charm towards her thought she had a relationship with him and that the recommendation was too severe as it was his first offence. Both the professionals recommended a supervision order. When the case appeared before the court the Bench took the word of the psychologist and psychiatrist and placed the boy on a supervision order under the Probation Department for two years. Within three months the boy was back in the Centre again for Grievous Bodily Harm. He had stabbed another man in an incident similar to the first. It was an even more serious offence as the victim was in intensive care and at the point of death for a week. When the boy appeared before the court he was given the Detention sentence. The residential staff could not help feeling that had their recommendations been carried out the second case would not have happened.

The following is a case where residential staff had to do the social case work which unfortunately was too late, and they were of the opinion that had it been done at the start the outcome might have been vastly different.

A fifteen and a half year old West Indian boy had been in this country for about six months and had a limited knowledge of English. He was brought before the Court for Unlawful Sexual Intercourse and being beyond Parental Control. He was admitted to an Observation and Assessment Centre. The boy manifested behaviour difficulties, physically attacking staff with chairs, fists and anything else which came to hand. Psychiatric oversight was given and medical tests suggested the boy had severe brain damage. During the time he was in the Centre he committed an offence Of Grievous Bodily Harm, he stabbed an Indian gentleman. The incidents of violence continued at the Centre and the boy was taken before the Court where an Unruly Certificate was issued and he was taken to a Remand Centre. At this time he was thoroughly confused. He found the warders difficult to understand and it was thought that his spirit was broken and he alleged he was badly treated. Eventually he was taken to the Crown Court and transferred to a secure psychiatric hospital. It was felt by staff that had there been different psychiatric provision at the start the boy would not have finished in a mental institution. The boy had an extended stay at the Centre and the staff were of the opinion that social casework could be regarded as an act of gross mismanagement. During his stay at the Centre little or nothing was done to establish anything about his past or present circumstances. The medical history of the boy was not established until very late in the case. One of the residential staff visited his home and found that social worker involvement left a lot to be desired. There were a number of early histories which were not common knowledge but were related to residential staff and due to the lack of social work involvement were not known to the field worker. The only social worker contact between the field worker and the boy was during the time he was in the residential establishment. Staff felt therefore that had the casework method been established as we understand it, that is, home visits and a full investigation the outcome might have been different.[12]

Residential Life with Children - Christopher Beedell

1. The situation is quite simply this; the staff have to give a great deal to the children in their care. NO person has an inexhaustible fund of love and concern, and thus no one can effectively survive in these circumstances unless he is replenished. Such replenishment of giving resources is thus an absolutely necessary condition of good residential work. It is not, in itself, enough, for even when it exists the love and concern deriving from it may still be misdirected or ineffectively used. Contrariwise no technical expertise, in itself, will suffice to meet the needs of the children, nor can it be humanly and reliably maintained without the existence of a tolerably well-balanced emotional economy i.e. where giving and receiving are in roughly equivalent proportions for a fair amount of the time. It becomes necessary, therefore, to look at the stresses and satisfactions arising in residential work in some detail.

2. Any purely advisory function is potentially powerful but inevitably limited. Its power is often dependent on the public availability of information, and there is a difficult balance to be maintained here between information being acquired more easily because it is confidential and information not being acted upon because it is not made public. The power of the Inspectorate is, of course, also dependent on the quality of people recruited to it. There is a particular difficulty for residential work here because it has not, in the past attracted many people with substantial academic qualifications. Since these are often, quite reasonably required of Inspectors there are comparatively few inspectors with adequate residential experience themselves (though this is changing of late). In addition the Civil Service as a whole is not renowned for the recruitment of qualified and experienced specialists, to any but its very specialised departments. Inspectors also have to work within the limits of the built in conservatism of all social institutions, a conservation which is particularly potent in those institutions, agencies and units dealing with painful and potentially dangerous areas of human behaviour.

Child care and the Growth of Love- J. Bowlby

3. Because of this type of behaviour and because of the intensely personal relationships necessary, it is widely recognised that house-parents must be given the choice of accepting or refusing a child. A warm personal relationship with tolerance of much difficult behaviour cannot be provided to order. Moreover, each pair of house-parents will find one sort of difficulty easier to handle than another. For these reasons the policy of organising groups of hostels, permitting each to be a little different has much to recommend it.

Residential Care Reviewed P.S.S.C. 1977

74. Encouragement should be given to heads of homes and staff to take sufficient breaks away from the home setting. Strains can build up and outlooks become narrow without the staff themselves being aware of what is happening. Kindly insistence may be necessary to help staff escape temporarily from inevitable pressures.

Residential Work with Children- R. Balbernie

6. The evidence available by 1952 as to casuality in the field of maladjustment was summarised by Schonnell.

   While the results obtained are suggestive for both diagnosis and treatment, it is very important that we should realise that each maladjusted child is a unique case produced by a varied set of interacting and cumulative forces. Many studies of maladjustment do not go deep enough. We need a combined case study approach, involving all the possible factors, and a psychoanalytic approach penetrating to the deeper workings of the mind and revealing the motives behind maladjustment.

7. Some maladjusted children will need a new primary reference group (a family alternative), but how many children will require what form of special educational treatment in the future is as yet almost impossible to forecast. It is important and urgent to study and obtain

more information about the patterns of need that exist. A special unit which would be a combination of a good children's home and a day special school, providing careful, individual, remedial experience, may be suitable in some cases; in some cases a treatment centre within a flexible children's village might be a more suitable form of provision, and so on.

8. There is a tendency in all statutory agencies to accept for treatment cases beyond the actual therapeutic capacity (the resources and skills available) of the unit just because these agencies are continually under very considerable pressure to take on more than they can manage.

   The fact that role clarification is in itself an extremely painful, personally demanding, and complex matter in this field needs to be recognized clearly as it profoundly affects morale. Unless each staff member's task is defined and he is backed properly within an authorising structured setting in the primary and secondary tasks which he must undertake, considerable motional tension and confusion will result.

10. Each person will be conscious of the contribution of his role and the clarity of his area of professional responsibility and aware of how this contributes to the effectiveness or clarity of all other roles in the enterprise.

    Any discrepancy between what is desirable and what is possible will be objectified and remain a matter of conscious concern as will the gap between the job that should ideally be done, and the job actually being done.

    Each person must be clear as to what is not his task (i.e. when he is moving inside or outside the boundaries of his primary task and what is being left undone when he moves outside it). It is important to be clear about what is not being done. Collusive obscurity and evasion of painful reality by muddle will adversely affect the morale of the organization and will lead into motivated resistance to essential clarification.

11. When structure and organization is not sound, role boundaries and

interfaces will be obscured and professional interaction processes become confused and this tends to heighten uncertainty and anxiety.

Exceptional Children- Lenhoff

4.   A child guidance clinic consists of a team of three- the psychiatrist, the psychologist and the psychiatric social worker. Occasionally there is added a trained psycho-therapist, who will treat the child according to the diagnosis of the psychiatrist. The psychiatrist should be a specialist in dealing with children. Many symptoms which in adults would be diagnosed as severe mental trouble must be recognised in a child as merely a phase: a stage in his emotional development. It is the job of the psychiatrist to be completely impartial and permissive so that the child will talk freely to him, knowing that what he says will not be divulged either to his parents or to others in authority. Only then, when the facts are sorted out, can diagnosis be made and treatment begin. Traditional schools are possessive about their pupils. Too many teachers, insufficiently trained in psychology, either condemn their 'difficult' pupils out of hand for 'naughtiness' or take an attitude of self-defence. Many of them are not child guidance clinic minded and feel that recommending a pupil for treatment at a clinic is a confession of their own failure which they are disinclined to make. It is essential that psychology should be a part of education if we are to overcome the attitude that the symptoms of emotional disturbance are 'merely naughtiness'.

12.   The psychiatric social worker assembles a complete history of the child's background and environment, his development and the situation in which he finds himself in relation to his parents and siblings. He or she must find out at what stage and how the development of the child went wrong. Then it must be decided how, if possible, the mother can be taught where the mistakes were made and how she herself can put things right.

Chapter 2

I am frequently stunned at the number of people who apply for work in residential establishments and are totally ignorant of what this work really entails. So many imagine it is purely bath, feed and bed. This view of the residential task is too often held by people who should know better. The general opinion seems to be that houseparent's are glorified domestics and gardeners and should be treated as such, consequently this side of the service has become something of a Cinderella.

I have tried to explain to potential staff what there were undertaking, some to their credit admit it was not what they imagined and decline the post. Others blandly say they understand, spend a few months in a post and then leave. Many young men and women who have trained as teachers and done a fair amount of practical work with children apply for a post in Children's Homes because they have been trained to work with children and want to do just that. Unfortunately all too often they have a very rude awakening. One such appointment I made is a typical of the reaction.

A young man, well qualified as a teacher, wanted a job working with children. During the course of his training he had worked in some dockland schools in several big cities. He assured the panel that he had a fair knowledge of the problems he would face and duly started work in a home for eighteen children. For the first week things were not too bad. The Officer in charge advised him on the best way to approach the children and was politely told that it was not necessary as he could manage. The Officer in charge decided it was time the new staff was 'baptised' and left him with the children. There was also a housemother on duty. Within an hour the Officer in charge was called in. The place was in uproar, children were fighting everywhere and the air was blue with obscenities. The housemother was trying to restore order and the new member of staff was standing white faced and shaking. His comment when things were quiet again was, "These are not children, they are animals". The fact was that he viewed child care like so many others and was not prepared to listen to the voice of experience. The new staff member stayed for three months gradually losing heart and face with the children. One of the older girls said to him one day, "You're too soft, get off your arse and do something". He lasted one week after that and in fact took a job as a labourer. To be fair to the young man, his training had been in classroom situations, but there are far too many cases of people being trained specifically for residential work and proving unable to cope with the work, mainly because they accept everything taught on a course as "Gospel". [13:14:15]

The following cases illustrate this point.

There was a young man who was Deputy in a Working Boys Hostel. He went on a two year course, and shortly after he returned the Officer in charge took another post elsewhere. The young man applied for the Officer in charge post and was appointed. His reports from the course had been excellent and the senior staff in administration thought he was a bright lad. His philosophy was 'let it all happen' and happen it did, so much so that the hostel had to close. He was then sent to a large children's home as Officer in charge where he followed the same pattern. He allowed children to 'express themselves'. They wandered in and out of the office at will and were even allowed to go into the safe. The situation went from bad to worse and at one point the children were literally climbing on to the roof of the house. About this time neighbours started to complain and the administration had to act. A discrepancy was found in the book keeping and the young man quietly left. Officers in charge in the area were called to the office and the situation was discussed. They were told that it had been an "experiment". One Officer in charge who had been frequently criticised for running a "tight ship" was asked to go into the home and clear up the mess- he did!

There was a boy in a Children's Home who had been taken into care for truanting and some minor offences but the staff did not see him as a great problem. He started at school and for a while attended regularly then started to truant again. The Officer in charge had words with him and warned him that if he continued to truant the consequences would be very unpleasant.

About this time a young man who had just completed a two year course was appointed as Deputy and did not think that the boy was being handled in the right way and started to collude with the boy in this truanting, which of course got considerably worse. Eventually that boy was sent to a Community School. A year or so later the boy visited the Children's Home and said to the Officer in charge, "If you had kicked my arse when I was here I would be home now, wouldn't I?" The Officer in charge admitted that he was right.

You must realise that these young men were genuine and really believed what they were doing was right. It is also a sad reflection on tutors who imagine they can build the next course on what they learn from the current one. There is only one way to learn residential work and that is by physical contact with the clients. Courses should supplement this knowledge. I know of tutors who reject the practical experience gained by students on placement and refer to various passages in books. Also if the students writes or says anything which the tutor disagrees with personally, then he or she is censured. The fact that it could be good care is often beside the point. My own opinion, based on my own experience is that there is room for everything in child care and that nothing should be rejected out of hand.[16]

I relate the case of a young man on an In Service Training Course. It so happened that the tutor and other students on the course went to the home he worked in for a visit. The next day the visit was a subject for a discussion among the students. The tutor opened the discussion by condemning nearly everything about the home and the way it was being run. When the young man protested that they were not being fair and that he could vouch for the fact that it was a happy home and that staff relationships were excellent, the tutor proceeded to quote from the books and made every effort to belittle him saying, "Well you are bound to defend it, aren't you, after all you work in the place". The whole business was related to the Officer in charge of the home who in turn told his senior. The matter was taken up with the senior tutor and it came to light that the tutor in question had never been in residential work and her only contact with homes had been through visits with students. This tutor was prepared to make a judgement on an establishment on the basis of a couple of hours knowledge and even worse, she was lecturing others on a subject she obviously knew nothing at all about. The tragedy was that staff with very little experience were accepting everything she said and would expect to be able to deal with the problem children using this tutor's theories as a guide and then wonder why they did not get the response predicted.

Fortunately not all tutors are the same. One on a Certificate of Qualification in Social Work course had a student on placement in a mixed adolescent home. The tutor visited her student and during a meeting with the Officer in charge she asked if it would be possible for the student to be given some responsibility in the Home. This home had some particularly difficult boys and girls and the Officer in charge told the tutor that it would be unwise to put a student in such a vulnerable position as some of the girls "would eat the student alive". The student to his credit agreed with the Officer in charge and said quite openly that he was glad he had taken the field work option because he would not be able to cope in a residential home. The tutor accepted his word and the matter was left. It was just as well as the lesson was driven home a short time later. It happened like this. One of the girls had a visit from her mother. It was a dark wet night. When it was time for the mother to go, the student offered to give her a lift and the girl asked if she could go also for the ride. She was told "Yes". When they returned the girl said the student had exposed himself to her.

The student, a married man with three children, was horrified at the accusation and protested his innocence. Fortunately for him the Officer in charge was wise to the ways of his charges and after a short but skilful investigation it was found that the student had felt warm in the car and had loosened his tie!!![17] Those who imagine a residential worker is not vulnerable take particular note, but more of that later.

I have talked to residential workers about their views on students doing placements in homes and the following is their view.

Courses do not take residential work seriously. It is a case of telling the student you have a five or six week placement, go in and enjoy it. You are there as an observer but don't upset them. Be careful what you do and say because it is difficult to get placements and we may want to use that home next year. The student then regards the placement as a break from college and a home as somewhere you can put a client while you get on with social work. Courses, even C.Q.S.W. (Certificate of Qualification in Social Work), lean towards fieldwork and the emphasis appears to be on the qualification for field workers and away from residential work. There is an abysmal lack of training for residential work; at the last count it was reckoned that around fourteen and a half percent of residential workers did not have any form of qualification. Even so it is wrong to think that because a person has a qualification that they are going to be able to cope in residential work. The intangibles of residential work cannot be taught over a desk, they have to be learned through practical experience and it is no use a person doing a few months in a home then going on a course and coming away with a qualification thinking they know all they need to know about being able to deal with the problems residential work presents.[17]

Students come into homes with preconceived ideas mainly that residential workers are hard on children and yet within a month of being there they are harder than the staff and have to be watched. Most students assume that staff must be ruling with an 'iron rod' because when they are left with the children they find it a very harrowing experience. The children are unruly, disruptive, disobedient and try their patience in many ways yet when the residential worker walks in order is restored in a matter of minutes. The student is often convinced that this control is achieved by violence towards the children which they have yet to see. When they find that there is none their frustration is complete and a lot of this frustration is generated by their own unwillingness to accept what the residential worker says.[15]

The fieldwork student seems to be dealing mainly with Acts of Parliament-Law and Casework methods. Other than voluntary care Section I, what act the child has been brought in under does not greatly affect the residential worker. They are presented with the 'body' a living, breathing, human being and they are expected to do something with it.

It is quite natural to want to befriend children but students tend to 'overact' often going to great lengths to try and form relationships. Although the student is acting with the best of intentions they fail to realise that to the children he/she is a stranger, 'an incomer' and to start asking a child about his family, friends, school, hobbies, etc. will only cause the reaction "Only been here five minutes and already he is pumping me" or, alternatively, a child will see an opportunity to manipulate and seize it. As time goes on and the relationship the student was trying for fails to develop, they start to play favourites, mainly with those who are forthcoming, frequently causing problems for the child with the rest of the group and/ or the staff. Students can, with the best of intentions, cause many difficult situations for staff. They themselves, have gone off duty when repercussions of their actions show and staff have to sort it out.

Let me quote a simple example.

A student was a placement in a Children's Home. Due to an acute shortage of staff he was far more involved than he probably would have been. It was breakfast time and the children were coming in to the dining room. They had been helping themselves to cereals, some of the fine dust from the bottom of one of them fell onto the floor. No one knew who did it and it was probably accidental anyway. However, the Officer in charge passing the door saw it and said nothing about it. The student came in and sat down followed by a twelve year old who sat near the patch of cereal dust. The student noticed the dust and said to the boy in a sharp voice, "What's that?"

"What's what?", said the boy. "That", said the student. "What?" said the boy. The boy turned his back on the student mumbling to himself. The Officer in charge saw and heard all this exchange. Later the student said to him, "What have you done to Billy, he is sulking and snarling at everyone?" The Officer in charge said, "I (with the emphasis on the I) have done nothing to Billy. He's been alright with me". The fact of the matter was that the boy saw himself being accused of something he had no knowledge of and he was the type who would sulk at the slightest injustice so staff had to put up with the boy's bad mood all day. I say this to Course tutors. " Residential work is a serious task, please treat it so". As a learning experience it would be better for a student to work as a member of staff and cover a duty rota just like other staff in a home. They will learn far more than just being there and wondering where they fit in. If possible let the student visit the home before the placement for a serious discussion. Students are not aware of the intensity of residential work and after a short time it shows. It would help them if tutors would make a point of going into this, because without a longer placement the student is on his way back to college just when he is beginning to learn what it is all about. Remember it is very hard work to maintain equilibrium in a home and help a student at the same time. Also, staff are human beings with human failings. They have troubles of their own and are not perfect; they can lose their tempers and get tired. The demands made on an Officer in charge are considerable and a student increases these demands. Please be reasonable. I have spoken to students on placement and they all said they would not like residential work. They all found the work too intense and were quite concerned at the number of disturbed children residential staff had to cope with. One student said he looked forward to the placement with some enthusiasm but as the weeks went by he found himself frightened to go into the home and was glad when his day was over and he could get away. He admitted that at the end of each day he felt completely drained and said he found it difficult to understand how the staff managed to keep up with the pressures.

A word to students about forming relationships. Don't try to force the pace, if children want to form a relationship with you they will do it in their own time. Let them make the pace. Just be with them quietly but be awake to the opening gambits for testing out. Watch for the manipulators and check what they say to you. You may think that you can assess children but let me assure you that they will have assessed you long before you start on them. They will know your weak spot and your tender places and it you are not honest enough with yourself to know them, then you are in for some very unpleasant shocks. Sometimes it helps to find out what 'nicknames' they have given to you, it often gives an insight into what they think of you. Do not take umbrage if you find out and it is not pleasant.

If you should be unfortunate and get a placement where there are practices which give you cause for genuine concern, then have a word with your tutor. If you think the Officer in charge is not aware of it, have a word with him or her. If you decide it is serious enough to be brought to the attention of the senior administrative officers then be sure of your facts and be able to prove what you are saying.

A word to Officers in charge and staff. The student is also human and it is more than likely that a residential home is a completely new experience for him/her and they will be very strange if they do not feel some apprehension about the prospect. Be sure of the role they are to play, it is useless to put them in a role and later condemn them for doing it too well. I remember one placement I did and when word got out that I had worked in an approved school I was used as a policeman. It was a well known Children's organisation with a series of house units around a square. I started the placement in a unit with quite a reasonable group of children but was soon moved to another unit where the children, so I was told, needed discipline and a firm hand. When I provided them it was intimated to me that a housemother in charge of another unit had complained that I was too strict and she did not agree with what I was doing. I wasn't knocking the children about. I found later that this woman had a more subtle approach to controlling her charges! If they misbehaved or offended her she used to make them sit in a bath of cold water until they repented! How is that for projection? Senior staff were aware of this practice and were very embarrassed when I told them I knew about it and how long it had been going on. Altogether not a very happy placement for me.

A student, before coming into social work, may have been a bricklayer, plumber, joiner etc. They do not come to you to rebuild that bit of wall, repair broken cisterns or refit the door locks or any of the jobs you reported to your authority six months previously. They come to you to learn something about residential work. They are not there to be given all the dirty work that staff try to avoid, and if there is a problem which you or your staff have not the courage to deal with then do not give it to the student. If you would like the student to try some problems and he agrees, then be fair and give as much background information as possible.

I asked a student if he would like to comment and this is what he said. "I was brought up in care and I thought I would be able to work with children in a residential setting easily. I also wanted to see if things had changed since I was a child. I am old enough to have seen something of life and I have worked for some years as a social work assistant. I think I have a good placement in this home. I've been here for a few months now and my respect for the staff and Mr ..., the Officer in Charge has grown considerably. I just don't know how residential staff do it. I have tried very hard to control the children like they do but I admit I can't. I had no idea that children were such skilled manipulators. I've had several salutary lessons while I've been here. Lessons I won't forget. I volunteered to stand in for a week while Mr and Mrs ... took a holiday. They had not been able to have a break because they had been short of staff. What a week that was. They hadn't been out of the home very long when the children started. They played up in a way I wouldn't have believed possible. I know one thing, I wouldn't have their job at any price. I was glad when they came back but I learned more in that week than in any other period of my placement. People criticise residential workers but they are not in any position to do so, at least not until they have done about six months in a home."

"I took two boys for a walk and one of them ran across the road in front of a car. It shook me and when I caught up with him I slapped him and he said to me, "Do that again, I like it." That remark made me think and I will never do it again. I couldn't understand why Mr ... handles this lad so carefully. I told him about the incident and he was very understanding and told me not to worry about it."

"Mr ... and I took a group of children out one day and a boy who was beside me told me that Mr ... had hit him. I took him to Mr ... and asked him to repeat this, which he did. "when was this", said Mr ... "You know", said the boy. "Two years ago when I threw the pan at you". That taught me a lot about manipulation. I think this is the sort of thing that causes antagonism between residential workers and field staff and students. I've discovered that children will tell you part of a story and if you don't go in to it fully you can cause a good deal of trouble and ill feeling. The tutors seem to imply that if residential staff can maintain order in the home then there must be something wrong and infer that we should watch for it. Let's be honest, we can all find something wrong if we look hard enough and I think the staff in this home are very good and are doing a very difficult job. I think there should be special courses for residential workers and it would have to be much more intense than ours and I would make acceptance conditional on having done at least twelve months with very disturbed or maladjusted children.

"One morning after breakfast I asked some of the children if they would like a game of cards just to occupy them while they were waiting to leave for school. One boy said Mr ... would not let them play cards so I asked him about it and it transpired that he had once told the children they couldn't play cards and read comics all at the same time. Another lesson in manipulation.

"I came very close to a confrontation with a fifteen year old girl. Mr ... stepped in just in time and when he went over the incident I realised it had been building up for weeks. Mr ... had been aware of it and had let it develop for my benefit knowing he could stop it before it got out of hand.

"Tell me" said the student, "who does the Officer in Charge go to if he wants help. I have seen residential staff treated in a way which has made me furious. If a child is a trouble maker the field worker is involved and the Officer in Charge is usually given plenty of advice which invariably is negative, but if a child interferes indecently with another child there seems to be a marked reluctance for anyone to be involved and it is left to the Officer in Charge. If he takes a course of action which proves right half a dozen or more claim the credit but if it proves wrong the Officer in Charge is regarded as useless or a fool because he didn't do something else. These people can't win.

"I used to be sceptical when I heard about children being brought to a home without information about their case, but I have now had personal experience of this and also the timing. I think field workers should consider the time they take a child to a home. Often staff are busy with other children and they can not stop to spend time with the newcomer, consequently the child feels rejected and it makes for a very bad start.

"I have attended several reviews or case conferences on children since coming here and if what I have witnessed is an indication of what goes on up and down the country it is about time they gave up and stopped wasting money. One I went to had about ten people present including a psychiatrist and a psychologist. The residential staff might just as well have not been there. Everything they said was brushed aside as if they had no contact with the child at all.[18] The "experts" seemed determined to pin some sort of maladjusted label on to this child. They spent about two hours discussing the case and nothing really concrete came out of it in the end. In my opinion and that of the staff this particular child wasn't mad he was just plain bad and all he needed was a smacked bottom. Finally the panel of experts told the staff what they thought they (the residential staff) should do then left, leaving them with the problem. One of the staff caught my eye, smiled and shrugged her shoulders. She told me afterwards that it was the usual pattern. She said, "These people come to the home and insult our intelligence. I wonder why we bother to do this job". I was bitterly annoyed and went up to my room to cool down which took some time When I think of the hours put in by these people and the pay they get for it and the way they are treated, it makes me boil".

In view of what I have just written I think it would be appropriate to give some examples of the kind of mentality which is prevalent among some of the children the residential worker has to deal with.

There was a particularly difficult 12 year old boy, staff had been saying for eighteen months that he needed a structured environment and a firm hand. However, he went on a day trip with his school. When they all returned the children made their own way home as it was only about five o'clock. This boy went to a house about 200 yards down the road and asked for a glass of milk. The lady who had answered the door knew he was from the Children's Home and refused the milk and closed the door. The boy pulled up all the plants in the garden before he made his way home.

A new housemother had been working in a family group home for about a week. She was surprised and pleased when a ten year old boy asked her if he could help her to set the table for the evening meal. It was 3 o'clock in the afternoon. The Housemother in Charge came in at half past and remarked on the table being set. The new staff related what had happened and said how pleased she was and what a nice little boy he was. The Housemother in Charge smiled and told her that the boy had been making a nuisance of himself the previous night while playing table tennis and in order to punish him the other children had confiscated the ball and the table setting was a ploy on his part to ensure that the others could not play table tennis before the evening meal and also he was not to blame as he had only helped a member of staff set the table.

"While I was running an Assessment Unit I had a housefather who was genuinely concerned about and had good relationships with all the children. He took a group out for a walk one afternoon, they returned with one boy holding a handkerchief to his eye. I looked enquiringly at the housefather who indicated that he wanted to speak to me privately. We went into the office and he said, "I will never cease to be appalled at the viciousness of these kids". He related what had happened. They had gone along quiet lanes and footpaths and he thinking to start a harmless game had shown them how to make a type of pea shooter using a piece of cow parsley stem with hawthorn flower buds for peas. The children played happily at this game for a time when he heard a shout of pain from behind and turned to see a boy with a flower bud sticking to his eye. Upon inspection he found that one of the "little dears" had made a slight modification to the game. One of them had discovered that hawthorn bushes had thorns as well as buds and if he took a thorn and pushed it in to a bud it made a "pea" that would really hurt. Needless to say the game was stopped.

A group of children I had, developed a way of making pretend gliding rockets using plastic drinking straws, cutting little slits in one end and fitting paper flights. Making and flying these gave them hours of pleasure. After a few days my wife was puzzled when some needles were missing from her sewing box. We soon found one of them sticking in the cheek of one of the boys. One of them had the "bright idea" of fitting the needle into the end of the rocket and throwing it. It was sticking right through the boy's cheek and I shudder to think what the outcome would have been if it had struck him in the eye.

One home I know had a brother and sister among the children. The boy was 13 and the girl 11. One night the children were going to bed and were romping in the beds as children do. After they had let off steam the housemother said. "come on, all in". While she said it she was pulling back the sheets of this particular girl's bed and it was fortunate that she did as there were several razor blades in the bed and with the children romping on the beds the sheets were badly cut. The Officer in Charge started an investigation and it was found that the girl's brother had put the blades in the bed. All he would say was that he hated his sister. The girl had to be moved for her own safety.

There was a boy of 14 who presented great behaviour problems in a home. He was an out and out bully and as devious as they come. He was transferred to an assessment unit where the cook was a young woman who went to a great deal of trouble to make food attractive for the children and to provide them with little surprises. She had saved her money and bought a small car which was her pride an joy. The boy asked if he could clean her car for her one day and the cook thought it was very good of him and agreed. When she saw the finished job she broke down and wept. He had cleaned the car with steel wool. The little blighter stood in front of her in wide eyed innocence and said, "Oh Miss, I thought I was doing you a favour". The Superintendent said to me latter, "That boy knows how to hurt".

Residential Life with Children – Christopher Beedell.

13. In children's units generally about 15% of staff have a specific qualification in residential child care and a further 10% to 15% have other qualifications, some not necessarily greatly relevant to the job but perhaps better than nothing.

    The residential worker is in direct contact with the child over a greater proportion of his life space and often over a larger total of life span.

    The residential worker is functionally closer to the parents in necessarily providing a larger part of the "parenting".

Exceptional Children - Lenhoff

14. Life in a community of maladjusted children opens the newcomers' eyes with frightening clarity to their own not fully developed personality. And the task of helping themselves, at the same time as facing and helping children whose symptoms and problems are often near their own, can be a terrifying experience.

15. During the initial period the new staff member may hate those who, already at ease with themselves and the work, try to help him towards an understanding of himself and the children. He feels that he must leave a platform of make believe strength and maturity and is afraid to reach out and face the challenge of his own readjustment. The continuation of the work on each child and the experience with every one of them project his own personality problems back to him with ruthless continuity. Many are afraid to make this step, when jobs are plentiful in which there is need to battle with one's self.

16. Children need freedom, but freedom within a framework which is strong but elastic, and it is no easy job to know just when to encourage, when to demand, when to ignore mistakes and when to tighten up. No amount of training can replace insight and flair in this delicate task.

17. Such people are extremely rare and if we are lucky enough to interest them in our particular field, they join the small circle of those satisfied to give a few years of their professional life to such work for others.

These latter may be intelligent men and women with love for children, willing to try out new ideas and perhaps already with some intellectual knowledge of the depth of their own reactions, motivations, anxieties, and aggressions. Whether they have already applied all this to themselves enough to be able to give out of their maturity of personality something to emotionally-disturbed children is another question.

Chapter 3

I feel very sorry for young people who are desperately looking for work these days but I feel bitterly annoyed when they give up twelve months or two years of their lives to attend pre-residential, home economic or some other such course in the hope of making a career for themselves. The application forms they complete for a post usually contain the same phrases, "I love children" or "old people" and then go on to list their placements – one or two days, at a most a week in a home. They have usually been tutored by disciples of the "love deprivation" theory and are under the misguided impression that all they need is kindness and consideration and success is assured. These young people are being totally misled. Is it any wonder that staffing residential homes is like a revolving door when they have no clear idea of what it really entails. Some of the children in care are nearly the same age and often physically bigger than they are or they will be verbally abused and may be physically attacked. Out of all the young people I have employed in homes only one remains and she is in a home for the aged. Three months is about as long as they stay.

A colleague of mine was invited to attend a lecture on such a course. The lecturer was quoting from an open text book in front of him and the students were hanging on to every word. Finally he asked for questions. None of the students spoke but not so my colleague. She had many years of residential experience and she began to question the theories quoted. The lecturer closed the book, stood up and left saying "Well, I'll leave you to discuss it amongst yourselves". If students have neither knowledge nor experience of the task then the tutor is on very safe ground for no one can argue. My colleague was never invited again.

I was talking to a residential worker some months ago employed in one of a group of homes on a campus. He told me that in one of the homes there was a slight, small housemother and all her 'children' were adolescents and when she censured them for bad behaviour the children would put her in the sink and just go on with what they were doing.

Residential workers are told that containment should be by relationships. If a child absconds it is implied that the staff of the home are failures because they had not formed the "proper relationship". New staff worry about this, though as they gain experience they learn that it is all pure theory and that containment is not always possible on that basis. Residential workers know if a child makes up his mind to run, short of putting him behind bars or chaining him to a wall there is nothing they can do about it or, if a "child" attacks them physically there is very little they can do about that either.

I must admit to being sceptical of residential workers who say they have never had a physical confrontation with a child. I do not mean a knock down, drag out fight but "I'm not f...... well doing it and you won't make me" confrontation. Let us be perfectly honest, there are bad residential workers just as there are bad field workers and I admit many confrontations should not happen but I do not subscribe to the theory that all confrontations can be avoided. Many "difficult" or "delinquent" children have every intention of forcing a confrontation and no matter how often staff try they find themselves in a position where they have to make a stand and face the prospect of physical violence and it is not a very pleasant thing to be faced by a physically mature six foot boy or girl of 17 or so who is determined to establish their physical superiority over you. I will say this, if you find yourself in this position and you back down you may as well hand in your notice for you will do no good with that child or any of the others because having seen one "beat you" they will all "have a go" and I do not care what the experts say.

It would be interesting to find out how many assaults on residential staff are recorded in the national statistics because it is my experience that Social Services Departments and authorities in general find it more expedient to pretend that incidents of this nature do not happen or that staff are at fault. When a member of staff is forced into a position where they have to defend themselves they literally take their career into their hands, because if they strike a child it is more than likely that they will be suspended or dismissed. Factories have been brought to a standstill by strike action because a foreman swore at a worker but in residential work "Thou shalt not kiss, cuddle or kick". Of course, according to those who dictate our lives in this work, you are allowed to use physical restraint, which means you can hold them until they calm down. Have you ever tried catching a tiger by the tail?

Let me quote some examples.

There was a particularly difficult twelve year old girl. It was agreed that due to her violent nature she should be assessed. She was placed in an Assessment Unit and for a week or two everything was alright. One evening the housemother was walking past the telephone which she was using and the girls language was obscene. The housemother told her to stop using such language and was told, "Mind you own f...... business, I'm talking to my friend". The housemother took the telephone from her and put it down on the rest. The girl threw herself at the housemother, split her lip and her cheek and also pulled out a good handful of hair. It took four members of staff to restrain the girl and when order was finally restored the officer in charge told the girl she would not be allowed to use the telephone again. Eventually the girl had to be sent to an establishment which would impose strict control.

There was the case of a twelve year old mixed parentage West Indian girl which was related to me by a woman who was a housemother at the time. The girl was so violent that the field worker was terrified of her. Residential staff had for some time been asking for her to be moved to a secure unit but without success. The girl was involved in some trouble whilst out one day, the police arrived and in the melee the girl dislocated the policewoman's jaw. She also put two girls from school into hospital, took on six skinheads and laid them all out. She was completely disruptive in the home and would fight anybody. A girl she knew was admitted to the same home and it was discovered that they had been responsible for burning down a school. The second girl used to hide cigarettes in her rectum. She was eventually placed on remand and her reaction was frightening. The social worker shook with fear. She was placed in a secure room for four days. Whilst in there she tore a bar from the window and the

Superintendent said she had ruined the cell. I would remind you that this was a twelve year old girl.

Whilst in the process of writing this book the "Daily Mail" has reported a case of a housemother being raped by three teenagers and I have since read several articles about residential work, questioning what goes on in homes and community schools. Also it makes the public aware of the conditions under which staff often work. Residential workers know that these reports are only the "tip of the iceberg". The Housemother admitted letting the "children" touch her breasts. Now some people might throw up their hands in horror but too many regard this as good child care or give it a fancy name- therapy. The incident did not surprise me one bit, how more housemothers are not raped is what surprises me.

I did a short spell in a well known closed unit whilst on one of my placements. In this unit was a housemother aged about twenty-three. There was also a boy of sixteen who abused staff continually. I was told about this boy and in the fullness of time he came my way and me being somewhat slight of stature he thought he was on safe ground and started his abuse. A minute later he was on his back and I advised him not to try it again or his next job would be picking his teeth up from the floor. From that moment I had absolutely no trouble with him or any other boy. The housemother approached him in a different manner. She was a "therapist" and short of actually copulating the boy did pretty well what he liked with that young woman, any sensible woman would have knocked his head off. While I was there the last case conference on the boy was held. Believe it or not there were twenty-one people there including psychologists and psychiatrists. The conference went on for three hours, the housemother relating in detail what the boy had done to her and how she interpreted his actions. If this was not enough the "experts" and "professionals" sat there nodding their heads wisely at this young woman's tale and the tales of abuse from other staff. The decision of all these people was, since everything had been tried without success, the only thing left was to send the boy home where he would get in trouble again and the police would send him to Borstal!! It was at this time that someone mentioned that I seemed to have formed a relationship with the boy and that he was always most polite to me. The Head of the Unit asked if I would like to comment as I had not said a word since the meeting started. I pointed out to them that they had not tried everything and they immediately started to relate all that had been done but before they got properly started I said, "Have you tried giving him a thrashing?" The silence was deafening. I related what had happened between the boy and myself and the meeting became an uproar. It occurred to me at this point that I was an outcast amongst these people. The boy was sent home next day and I went to another unit in the school.

In view of what I have said in the last few pages and what I intend to say, it might be of some use to the reader to hear what some of the "experts" offer in the way of advice.

In our view immediate suppression of difficult behaviour regardless of the circumstances in which it occurs is unlikely to help children. A child might be better helped if such behaviour, which is often a symptom of underlying disturbance, is allowed to manifest itself. He may need to give overt expression to his feelings in difficult and hostile behaviour and also verbal abuse.

Another. A therapeutic environment is one in which informal communication is encouraged, where there is understanding and tolerance of deviant behaviour where the child has opportunity to express symptoms of his disturbance.

And again. A very deprived and disturbed child is unlikely to benefit from help unless there are some underlying controls. However, in our experience, in a residential establishment where the child's needs are properly understood and there is good communication between staff and child, relationships can develop between them which obviate the need for external controls. (Care and Treatment in a planned environment).

In other words, "Prepare to be a good doormat or you are no use in this work".

Another quotation. "Rewards for bad behaviour greatly increase the possibility of going on to worse behaviour".

Chapter 4

Y ou will no doubt have read or heard about the experiment performed on rats in a maze. The rat receives an electric shock when it goes down the wrong passage and gets a reward of food when it goes down the right passage and performs according to the experimenter's wishes (learned behaviour). So why in heavens name are we continually exhorted to reward bad behaviour in children. Of all the children I have dealt with, not counting those abandoned or orphaned, only a very small percentage could be genuinely described as being mentally or emotionally disturbed.

There was an eleven year old girl who had been labelled brain damaged. Her father was dead and her mother had angina. The child manipulated her mother to the point of a heart attack. Whilst in a home she proved very violent towards other children. A request to move her chair in the dining room, culminated in her throwing a jug through the television screen. She was sent upstairs to calm down. A housemother came on duty and being ignorant of the incident went to call the girl for a meal. She walked out of the room in front of the girl and was pushed downstairs. The result was an injury to her knee and hip which left her with a permanent limp, and she is now out of the work. Secure provision had been asked for, before and after the incident. Eventually she was sent to an assessment unit where she wrecked the furniture and was finally removed to a secure remand home.

Staff in homes do not only face the prospect of violence from their charges, but also from parents or relatives and the prospect is often more alarming as this type or person often brings help.

A personal friend of mine who is a senior housemother, had occasion to keep a girl in for one night for stealing and lying. The girl's mother lived round the corner from the home. She was thirty-six years old, living with and pregnant by a seventeen year old boy who was in the care of the Local Authority. The field worker was aware of this and condoned it. The girl got one of the other women to take a letter round to the mother, telling her a pack of lies and that the housemother would not let her go out. The mother came to the house with three teenage girl helpers. She started pushing the housemother around and using obscene language. The housemother knew the three girls who had been in her care some years before, so she chased them and started to defend herself against the mother. The mother then left after telling her not to go out at night as she would be waiting for her with a bottle of acid.

I said earlier that in this work you walk a razor's edge in a maze and that you would get little or no help. The following may serve to illustrate the point.

There was a man who was Superintendent of a large home in the North. In the home was a family of five children. Mother and father were not married and the father had a history of violence. He was released from prison after serving a sentence for grievous bodily harm, and he and his cohabitee made straight for the home and demanded the children. The field worker was there at the time and she had been made aware of the father's intentions. The staff on duty told the man that under the law they could not let him take the children, where upon he started to abuse and threaten them. The staff were afraid as they knew his reputation and as the situation was getting out of hand they called the Superintendent, who was off duty at the time. When the Superintendent arrived, the man threatened what he would do if his children were not handed over there and then. (at this point the field worker got into her car and drove off). One word led to another and ended with the Superintendent physically putting the man off the premises. The man then went to the office and complained that he and his cohabitee had been attacked by the Superintendent, and they of course had not done anything. The same people told the story to the local newspaper. The first the Superintendent knew of it all, was when the editor of the paper telephoned and told him what they had been told, and stated his intention of printing the story. The Superintendent told him to go ahead and print and he would sue them. They obviously thought better of it as the story was never printed. However, the Superintendent was called before seniors and Committee members to answer accusations which had been made. He soon realised that it was a full investigation and that he was in the hot seat. Among other things, he pointed out to them that they had taken the children into care not him, and that he had not only to defend himself, but the staff as well and that they should be aware of the man's record. The Superintendent was reprimanded and told not to let it happen again. The field worker on the case made no offer to support and obviously the seniors and the authority did not want any press reports, for that would have meant explanations!! Needless to say the Superintendent looked for another authority to work for and I hope he has found one that will give him some support, though I doubt it. [19:20:26]

It would be more useful if those who order our lives both at local and national level knew something about residential work, for as things stand at the present time there are too many theorists telling too few practitioners what to do. At local level, policies and methods of practice are decided by bus drivers; shopkeepers etc. who have probably spent at most a few odd hours in residential homes either for children, old people or mentally handicapped persons, and it would be interesting to know how many directors of social services have any real residential experience.

It is very often the residential worker who is seen to be the villain, keeping the children, and not the fieldworker or the local authority, though sometimes it does work out well as in the following case.

There was a family of five in care. They had been under a lot of pressure; their father was a big, violent man and had been in prison for grievous bodily harm. The children had seen him knock mother about on many occasions causing her to take an overdose. The children's school teacher had asked if she could take them out which pleased the housemother.

The father heard about this and went round to the home demanding the children back and, of course, threatening what he would do to the housemother if she let the teacher take them out again. When he was requested to contribute towards the children's care, he went down to the office, threatened the clerk and would have nothing to do with the office. After some weeks he realised that the housemother was genuinely concerned about the welfare of his children and so he brought money to the home regularly.

There is no one more alone than the residential worker with a crisis on his/her hands. In crisis situations the residential worker has just a few seconds in which to decide on a course of action. If he/she makes the wrong decision it may well mean he/she is no longer in a position to control the group. It is easy to see what he/she should have done after an incident, and it is even easier for others to say what should have been done, but whatever the residential worker thinks or others say, it is that particular time which counts because the residential worker has to do something.

There was a girl of twelve in a home, two of her sisters had absconded from approved school. They had made their way to the home and hid in a derelict car in the grounds. There were two housemothers on duty, but neither was aware of this. The first indication the staff had of anything amiss, was when they caught the child creeping down the fire escape with blankets and food. The staff stopped her whereupon she picked up a bottle of milk and went for them with it. The staff ran away and locked themselves away in the office until she calmed down. The girl was only about five feet tall and her respect for the staff left a lot to be desired. The two staff left soon after as they found they could no longer control the other children who had witnessed the whole incident. The Senior Housemother said, "You should have taken the milk from her and, if necessary, poured it over her head, then brought the sisters in, given them a meal and called the school".

A field worker and a residential colleague had agreed that a rather difficult seventeen year old girl was in need of a short spell of strict discipline. In good faith the field worker arranged for a remand home to take her for five or six weeks. The particular remand home had a points system for privileges. The staff of the remand home were having quite a difficult time with the girl. However she stormed into the Superintendent's office and said, "Hey you, what the f...... hell do you mean by putting me on Grade I". The Superintendent replied quite timidly, "Well you haven't been very co-operative have you?" " Listen you", she said, "you get me on Grade IV or I'll really give you some trouble". She was duly put on Grade IV. Two days later she assaulted a much smaller girl giving her a very severe beating. The Superintendent put the girl who had been assaulted into a secure room and told staff it was for her own protection!! When the girl went back to the Children's Home the fieldworker and her residential colleague found she was worse than when she had left and the staff had the hopeless task of trying to control her. Eventually she had to be placed in a Community school.

Remember what I said about senior staff expecting others to do what they cannot or will not do themselves. In the above case the junior staff were obviously placed in an impossible position, and one could hardly blame them for not bothering.

The following is a case where the Officer in Charge literally found herself very much alone, before and after an incident. A seventeen year old girl was placed in an Adolescent Girl's Unit and she was known to be violent. The Officer in Charge though not happy about the prospect and being short of staff said she would do what she could. Over a period of days the girl made some minor skirmishes which made staff realise that sooner or later one of them would have to face an attack. The girl absconded and was returned by the police after a few days. They indicated their disgust at what she had been up to with some immigrant men in derelict property. When the police are shocked it must be bad! The Officer in Charge sensed trouble after the girl had been back a few hours. She telephoned the area officer, the senior social worker and the girl's social worker and told them in turn of her fears but not one showed interest. As the fieldworkers were on strike, they were not concerned about what happened after 5p.m. She was given the telephone number of the duty doctor. As she suspected it happened that same night when she was on duty alone. The girl started to abuse her and when she remonstrated with her, the girl picked up a knife from the table and attacked her with it. After a struggle the Officer in Charge managed to take the knife from her and get the girl's arm up her back. By this time she had the girl on the floor. This went on for about twenty minutes with the girl mouthing obscenities and threatening what she would do and the Officer in Charge trying to calm her down. The Officer in Charge eventually got one of the other girls to ring the police who came and took the girl to the cells.

A case conference was called the next day and the very people who had shown such lack of interest, told the Officer in Charge how distressed they were that the girl should be subjected to the traumatic experience of having to spend the night in a cell!! No mention was made of what the outcome would have been if the Officer in Charge had been unable to get the knife from the girl, or had one of the other girls decided to assist in the attack. This Officer in Charge is still in the work and said she has been surprised how her prestige has gone up with the girls. She admits she has never had such peace or obedience from her charges.

I have said a residential worker is alone when such incidents occur; this is no exaggeration even when other staff are present. If you are the one the child has decided to challenge and if you want to avoid losing control of your group, then it is likely you will be left with no alternative.

I found myself in such a position twice whilst in residential work. The first was in a senior boy's approved school. I was on duty alone in a unit where there was a boy of eighteen, six feet tall, big of stature and a bully of the worst kind. He ran a gang in the school and terrorised all the boys. The boys who did not do as he wanted were beaten up. The Headmaster was aware of this and made no effort to do anything about it. I saw a result of the gang beating once, and I assure you it was not very pleasant. This particular night I was doing some work in the unit office and among other activities there was a game of table tennis in progress. I suddenly sensed something was wrong and went to see what was happening. This particular boy had a bat in his hand and was telling another boy to play with him. The rest of the boys had stopped what they were doing and were looking very sullen. I realised he had taken a bat from one of the boys who had been playing. I took the bat from him and gave it back to the original player and told him to carry on. He was very reluctant understandably, as he was afraid of reprisals. The bully started to make abusive remarks to me and threatened what he and his gang would do to me. I took a chance. I said, "Right son, you and I will go to the barn and whoever walks back is the better man. If you walk back I will leave". He declined the offer and I had little trouble with him afterwards, and I became a friend of all the boys.

The strange thing was, I had told all the boys on several occasions that if they stood together against this bully, he would not have a chance against them.

The second incident was in a junior approved school. I had worked hard for two years on a group of boys and besides this I was also running a Reception/ Assessment Unit. I was told we would be getting a boy of fourteen who had terrorised every teacher he had been put with. This had been reported in the newspapers and we were told that the boy carried paper cuttings around with him – his status symbol. The first contact I had with him was when I went to pick up the boys from the school block. I always liked to keep new boys close to me for a while until I got some idea what to expect from them. However, he came out with the other boys and started to walk away. I asked where he was going and he gave me a look of disdain and said, "The Office". I said "Get into line with the other boys and I will tell you when you can go to the office". I had every intention of sending him to the office, but with another boy who I knew would see he got there and back. He rushed at me and aimed a punch. I tripped him and told him to behave himself and get into line. All this time every boy in the school and the duty staff were watching him and waiting the outcome. He started cursing me, tore off his jacket and threw himself at me again. While we were struggling, my housefather started to interfere. I asked him to stay out of it as I would have to handle the boy. Eventually, I put him on his back and told him of the consequences of a further attack. Whilst this was going on, one of my regular boys had gone to get the Headmaster. When he arrived I apologised for what had happened and he said, quite cheerfully, "That's alright, Mr Taylor it took four policemen to get him into school". I took the boys across to the unit and this boy refused to come in. I had warned him that if he came into my unit he would do as he was told and behave himself. My wife said the evening meal was ready, and I went to tell him to come and get it. The headmaster was with him, he refused to come and said he would abscond. "Alright", said the headmaster, "I'll give you half an hour's start". A few weeks later a colleague met a man from another school where this boy had been sent. He told my colleague about having this boy and that he was no trouble, and that he could not see what all the fuss was about as they had been given reports of this boy being violent. My colleague said "No, if Gordon Taylor hadn't sorted it out you would have had it to do".

Many people reading this may get an impression that I am in favour of violence from staff, but I assure you that I am not. In no circumstances would I condone brutality, but I have said that I believe there is room for everything in child care, and I firmly believe that corporal punishment has a place. I know some who read this will disagree but I look at the other side of the coin and what I am about to relate happens regularly.

An Officer in Charge adheres strictly to the letter of the law. No physical punishment, yet he will arrange it so that any child he thinks needs a smack is put with a member of staff he knows will do it. Alternatively, it will be something far more insidious and damaging- mental manipulation or to put it bluntly – mental sadism. It leaves no visible marks and the effects do not show for some time. Eventually, after judicious manipulation at case conferences the child is moved on and some other residential worker finds they have a completely disturbed child on their hands, with little or no chance of doing anything about it. The child, if young, may have no idea of what has been happening.

Bear in mind that this sort of practice is engaged in by people who have no real idea of the damage that they are doing. – irreparable damage. It is my experience that this practice is motivated by frustration due to the lack of support and understanding from seniors and authorities, and it is my contention that it is a manifestation of the aggression, albeit misplaced, which they feel for their seniors. It must be appreciated that these people can put their hands on their hearts and say with all honesty "I would never strike a child" and the 'enlightened ones' will smile at people like me and say, "There you are, we are right, that is the way it should be done". Psychologists tell us that frustration produces aggression and there is plenty of evidence to support this. Surely if this holds good for children in care, it also holds good for staff.

A colleague of mine attended a lecture when he was a student. The man giving the lecture was a well known personality in the child care field, and having written several books on the subject, is considered one of the experts.

Towards the end of the lecture the Senior Tutor said to my colleague, "what do you think of him?" My friend replied, "That man is a fool". The lecture finished and the lecturer started to leave. As he reached the door he turned to the class and said, "There is one thing I forgot. Remember this is the best psychology", and he held up a clenched fist!

We are currently being bombarded by demands for more training for residential and field workers. I am all for training but what kind? Too many people are coming from courses with bizarre ideas of residential care due to the 'deprivation theorists'. They identify so strongly with the client they end up defending the very problem they are employed to cure.

There was a student who did very well on a placement in an approved school. He dazzled everyone with his theories. When the course finished he took a job in a school and impressed the headmaster to the extent that he was put in charge of a unit. Other staff soon became heartily sick of the bad behaviour of boys from his unit as it was also affecting their boys. This young man justified bad behaviour by quoting psychology. One evening a staff member, off duty, was passing this unit and heard a terrific noise coming from it. He went in to investigate and found all the boys masturbating each other. He looked around the unit for this particular young man without success. At a staff meeting which was called, this young man, as usual tried to justify this incident but unfortunately for him, his excuses fell flat. He eventually left and the unit felt the effects for several years when it was agreed to run it down and start again with new staff. I understand that this young man was employed by another authority, believe it or not, as a child care adviser.

There was a man who sold two lucrative businesses to take up residential work and went to work in an approved school. He worked there for eight years, all the staff agreed he knew his job and had a great respect for his ability. He was a disciplinarian, but very just and had only ever struck two boys in the time he had been there; once to prevent a boy hurting himself and the second when a big boy was attacking a new member of staff. The school got a new headmaster with several degrees and who was one of the scientific child care disciples. The new headmaster did not agree with the housemaster's methods in spite of the fact that his ability and success were obvious to all. He started to make life difficult for the housemaster. He banned smoking, yet bribed boys with cigarettes to spy on staff. Nothing that the housemaster did suited the headmaster, who also turned his attention to the housemaster's wife and children and made life unbearable for them. Staff were of the opinion that the headmaster was jealous of the housemaster's ability and in view of the head's attitude discipline crumbled. The housemaster left the work and went back to business. These are brief details of downright incompetence which went on for quite some time. I might add incompetence, which is not peculiar to residential work. I understand this particular headmaster was, and for all I know still is employed by an authority as a Councillor in Child Care.

How long is residential work going to be bedevilled by these sorts of fools? There is no doubt the "Love and Deprivation" theorists have an awful lot to answer for.

Exceptional Children – Lenhoff

19. Managing committees or sub-committees for special schools are always answerable to some other superior body, and many of their members are afraid of public opinion and play for safety. Few of them have sufficient specialized knowledge to defend their ideas when necessary. These committees rarely look for outstanding people with strong individuality, drive and conviction to be heads of their schools, but rather for some trustworthy person prepared to toe the line set by the committee of the period, though certainly there are exceptions as in everything.

Residential Life with Children – Christopher Beedell 1970.

20. The appointment of trained and skilled residential workers to senior agency posts would do much to remedy this situation. "Though there is a shortage of suitable people there is a similar need for consultative service to residential units directed, not so much towards psychiatric problems (though that too is often needed) as towards providing a service for heads of units in particular".

21. I have already stated that I feel that all social agencies stand at the front door of the problem of moral breakdown and confusion in a society. This danger bears repeating. They are at the watershed of the fragmentation and projection of moral responsibility in the communities in which they exist and so are themselves at risk. Any agency which blindly colludes with the projection or responsibility from the community context will find itself unable to define or carry out its primary task. Such loss of reality within an agency (usually associated with a combination of weak leadership and organizational confusion) means a loss of a sense of solid achievement in role in all areas and so the morale and integrity of workers is depressed. This causes anxiety and guilt and workers feel it is either 'my fault' or 'theirs' or 'ours'. The actual circumstances and reality are, in fact, painful and are repressed and become a troublesome shadow and so communication about realities breaks down.

26. Groups of those directly involved in the actual work situation and practical problems working together on these are essential if <u>reality is not to be lost in this field.</u> The harmful collusive and schizoid splitting and fragmentation of this work begins unobtrusively where leadership fails and becomes depersonalized and dissociated with the reality and responsibility for actual task performance. There are many well meaning conscious citizens who willingly collude in this on committees in wanting, for apparently the best motives, a finger in the organizational pie without the responsibility of a legitimate role. Such bodies have an important task but require to be selected for their actual necessity and value, their experience and skill in understanding and facilitating the performance of the task of the enterprise and as useful resources, and with their own specific task as a body clearly defined. Sometimes, however, incompetents are appointed. These made the best scapegoats. A confused committee is a good cover for weak leadership and symptom of it. If the management body does not realistically define its own primary task and its limited area of actual responsibility in relation to the task of the enterprise (and if leadership is weak) other leadership roles may be trespassed on, diminished, and demoralized.

Chapter 5

T reatment- therapy- structured environment, these terms roll off the tongues of the "enlightened ones", reports and recommendations for children have an excess of these and similar terms. Students in this work are taught and encouraged to use them and with the continual brain washing, see themselves as ministering angels caring for the sick, fluttering about, soothing fevered brows as though the problems presented in this work can be cured by soft words and a bandage. [23]

The dictionary explanation is worth looking at:

Treatment- dealing with or behaving towards person or thing, (method of) treating patient or disease.

Therapeutic- of healing of disease, curative, - therapeutics- branch of medicine concerned with remedial treatment of disease. Therapy – curative treatment.

These terms have definite medical connotations and far too many people in this work see themselves in this light. One can almost see the saintly aura surrounding these workers and what is worse, they will use such terms to cloud their lack of ability or unwillingness to face up to hard facts. I read in a Social Work magazine and I quote, "he disputed the growing tendency to 'treat' (almost in the medical model)[23] when youngsters should have a right to be responsible and accept 'punishment'. Misguided treatment is the worst form of brutality." I could not agree more. I am also very critical of the use of these terms and their misguided interpretation.

A fieldworker friend of mine has a boy in a Community School and from the following story which he related it would seem that the Headmaster is suffering from the latest syndrome – allowing children to attend their review. The boy had absconded, broken into some premises and done a considerable amount of damage. My friend attended the review and asked where the boy was. The Headmaster said, "Oh, he doesn't want to come this time?" When the review was over my friend asked to see the boy and was told that he did not want to see his social worker. My friend said, "I'm sorry but I insist on seeing the boy." The headmaster replied, "Well you have a legal right to see him so I can't stop you." The implication here is that the Headmaster would have prevented the social worker from seeing the boy if he had been able. [39]

My friend was not in a very good frame of mind towards these particular residential workers when he related the story to me and I had every sympathy with him. I have grave doubts about the above practice and this incident only serves to crystallise them. If staff are going to adopt this practice then they should be consistent. If the child wishes to attend their review, then it should be made quite plain to them that they will attend good or bad. Staff do the child and society an injustice by letting the child hear only the good things about themselves and allowing them to opt out when they know they have done wrong and are about to be confronted with it. If we are going to prepare children for life when they leave care, then they should be made aware that society demands certain things and retribution for transgression is one of them. I think some of the examples I have already related, demonstrate what happens when children are allowed to imagine they have not broken the law. Both residential and field workers forget that they have a duty to society, the people they serve and who pay their salaries. I also am of the opinion that part of our duty is to co-operate with the police and not work against them in shielding law breakers.[39]

A seventeen year old girl was having an affair with a teacher in a school she was attending. The Headmaster found out and the girl was moved to another school. The teacher was married and the girl continued to go and stay with him when his wife was away. She told the Officer in Charge of the Home, that the teacher had said that he could get her a job as a model and asked if she could use the home as a base. The Officer in Charge questioned her very carefully about the job and discovered that it was a job as a pornographic model. She told the girl that if she wished to ruin her life that way, she would be better to find lodgings. The Officer in Charge told the girl's fieldworker who said, "Well girls do that sort of thing these days" and left it at that. What should have been done was to inform the police that the man was recruiting young girls for pornography; the girls name could have been kept out of it. As it was nothing was done and so by implication the social worker was condoning a disgusting form of law breaking.[24:75]

A woman I know who has had many years experience in residential work, was working in a children's home and became suspicious of one of the housefathers when she heard the children refer to bath time with him as "tummy tickle time". After patiently watching over a period of weeks she finally caught him in a homosexual act with one of the children. Her concern for the children dictated that she should report the matter to her senior. The Principal Officer she spoke to was a woman and when she heard the story told by the Housemother said that she was a "dirty minded, frustrated woman". (The Housemother had recently been divorced.) She realised then that nothing would be done and as she did not feel able to continue under such circumstances she left and took a post elsewhere. She heard from an ex-colleague some months later that both the Housefather and the Principal Officer had been dismissed. She was told that the Principal Officer had been found to be a lesbian. As far as she was aware the police had not been involved. I have great sympathy for the police in trying to deal with the young delinquents and criminals under the present system. If a child in care is apprehended for a criminal act, they realise they are virtually helpless because as the child is in care, there is nothing they can do other than leave it to the Social Services, who more often than not do nothing.

Senior Officers and those who dictate policy refuse to believe that children are capable of reasoning and have the guile to take advantage of woolly minded legislation which allows them to capitalise on the emotions of a closed minded section of society. Too many people who are in a position to do something about it collude with the children and protect them from the law.

I have a friend who is a magistrate. One evening when I met him he was in a roaring temper. When I asked him what the trouble was he related the following story.

He had been on the Bench that morning. A boy had appeared before him accompanied by his social worker. The boy had a string of offences although this would not have come to light at all if it had not been for a chance remark by the social worker, which caused the magistrate to ask some very pointed questions regarding the case. The result was that the Bench realised that the fieldworker had been deliberately lying to protect her client. My friend said to me, "Don't these people realise that when they are in Court they are officers of that Court and what is more, by such behaviour they encourage children to lie and manipulate. Such people should not be allowed near children".

In a Home I know there was a seventeen year old girl who was causing a lot of trouble, staying out late, getting drunk and encouraging dubious men to follow her home. At a review the Housemother said she needed support from the fieldworker to stop it, as men were banging on the doors and windows and frightening the younger children. A Senior Fieldworker saw the girl when the Housemother was present and told her that she was of age and could sleep around if she wanted to. At a review on the girl some weeks later, this same man was complaining that the girl was in constant trouble and wanted to know why the Housemother was not controlling her! [25:75]

Residential workers are subjected to abuse, condemnation, vilification and invective from all sides including 'clients'. I spoke to an Officer in Charge and put this to him. He said, "If I thought I was only here to be a receptacle for abuse I would get out, but I admit it is happening to a degree which gives rise for concern".

While I do not think residential workers have been paid for what they do, in my talks with them the last thing they spoke of was money. The main complaints were conditions and the abuse they were expected to put up with (Those who wonder why staff turnover is so great take note.)

An Officer in Charge of an Adolescent Girls Hostel had occasion to call in the fieldworker of one of the girls. The girl had been creating trouble and had kicked the Officer in Charge in the stomach. What few sanctions were allowed were brought to bear, including a ban on smoking. The fieldworker duly arrived and spoke to the girl alone. When he had finished he said to the

Officer in Charge, "It's quite simple, she will behave if you let her do as she likes". The officer in Charge replied, "What you mean is I should submit to whatever this girl wishes to do to me then you won't have to do anything positive". If an attack of this nature or one with a knife took place in public, the attacker would find himself/ herself on a very serious charge, but as the law stands the attacker is in the care of the Local Authority so nothing is done.

I watched a programme on television some months ago. It was from Manchester and it dealt with adolescents who had all been in trouble with the law and some had been in Borstal. There was a fieldworker with them and he was defending their way of life. When questioned by the interviewer he used the word "deprived" several times and talked about the conditions in which they had grown up. The interviewer turned to one of the young men who admitted threatening people to obtain money, and asked him why he did it. The young man replied, "Well, we are deprived of things". "What things" he was asked. "Well things", said the young man. It was obvious even to the most inept that he was on the deprivation wagon and that the fieldworker was colluding with all of them.

The point I would like to make is that we are all deprived to some extent. There are many things we would like but we do not all resort to violence against the helpless to obtain them. If we accept the laid down criteria none of us should be in this work. Deprivation is relative. Old people are beaten up and robbed, a little boy is deliberately murdered whilst delivering papers, a young woman is brutally murdered whilst walking her dog, a security guard is killed for £5000. I would remind people who read this that these callous thugs of today were the deprived, disturbed, misunderstood little dears of yesterday, nurtured in the bosom of the "Love, deprivation theorists" who have become contemptuous of the cries of those who live in fear and have become so arrogant that they have lost touch with reality.

It is all very well for the media to run programmes/ articles on this work, but you can only expect carefully edited versions calculated to arouse the emotions of the public but I do not accept it all without question. I was born and grew up in a poor part of Liverpool. I know what it is like to have no sheets on the bed and I know what it is like to go without. If all the teachings mean anything then I should be a master criminal at the present time.[27]

Another programme I watched "Elton House" dealt with violent psychiatric cases. Inmates were assessed on a points system, food and home leave being withheld for non compliance with the programme worked out for them. Complaints were voiced that N.U.P.E (National Union of Public Employees) had refused to allow their members to work there, also some suppliers had "blacked" the place. The psychiatrist in charge was pleading his case and talking about the success they were having. Nobody mentioned that the points system was thrown out of child care years ago and that we are not allowed to withhold food, and that residential workers have very little say in the matter of home leave. What are these measures? Only a form of punishment which is frowned upon today and I am still waiting to hear the howls of indignation from the "enlightened ones".

Speaking of psychiatrists reminds me of one I met whilst in residential work and this case is not unusual as many workers will know.

I was working in a Senior Boys Approved School and the Headmaster decided that we should have a psychiatrist in regular attendance. It was duly arranged that one should attend two evenings a week and we were asked to decide which boys should see him. Six of the boys in my charge were chosen. I noticed after a few visits that all the boys returned to the Unit in very good humour. I found out why when the first psychiatric reports were received. I could hardy believe my eyes when I read them. They might have been totally different boys from the ones I knew. I spoke to the psychiatrist about them and he assured me that his assessment was correct in the light if his interviews with the boys. I set out to find out how he arrived at such conclusions.

This involved some very diplomatic questioning of the boys when they returned from their weekly visits and it was not long before I discovered they were telling the psychiatrist the most outrageous stories about themselves and he was believing it all. When I was absolutely sure I went to see him and told him what was going on. He steadfastly refused to believe that the boys would do such a thing and so the game continued. I asked the boys why they did it.

Their reply was, "He wants to find something wrong with us so we're only helping him, besides he gives us cigarettes and it keeps him happy".[28:29]

Residential workers are continually being told what they cannot do. I would suggest that it would be more helpful if they were told what they can do. As I see it residential workers are in a limbo. There is no one more alone than the residential worker with a crisis on his/her hands. If a child attacks and they ring a senior, any damage will be done before the senior can get there (always assuming the senior was interested) because the worker must do something but there is nothing to protect him in law. There is a totally negative attitude on the part of authorities in general and I am of the opinion that the ignorance of policy makers is a major factor. They have listened to the so called experts telling them what is good child care. (He is king of the country of the blind who has one eye.) If a child sets out to attack you, then you are left with no alternative but to defend yourself, yet if you do strike a child and he/she runs away and tells someone you struck him, you do not have a leg to stand on because society will believe the child first. I am sure that policy makers close their eyes to the vulnerability of staff in such circumstances. It is naïve and stupid to say no children are bad or wicked and it is equally stupid to say all children are bad. Many of the children who get into care are very skilled at lying and manipulating for their own ends and are not above turning an innocent happening into a major incident to further their own ends or out of sheer spite to damage a member of staff.

Children can go sledging, skateboarding, roller skating etc. and get bruised in the process and some are then not above absconding and showing their bruises and accusing staff of causing them. I have seen this happen on several occasions and I am continually amazed at the stupid closed minded attitude of some seniors towards this. There was a case of a young Deputy in a children's home. He was a sensible young man and had learned his trade well. Also in this home was a fourteen year old boy – a real criminal in the making. A bully, devious and prone to lead other boys in the home into criminal acts. This boy encouraged another boy to support him in accusing the Deputy of beating them up and they showed bruises to support their accusations. I was brought into it by the fieldworker. I went to the Home and acquainted the Officer in Charge with the situation. He vehemently denied all charges against his Deputy and maintained that it was completely out of character for the Deputy to strike a child. The Deputy also denied having struck the boys. As the matter had been brought to my attention by the fieldworker who left me in no doubt that she expected something to be done about it, I was left with no alternative but to start an investigation. Meanwhile the two boys were moved to an assessment unit. The Officer in Charge of the Family Group Home told me that two days prior to the accusation having been made, they had returned with the children from holiday and the last day had been spent surfing. I leave you to imagine how much bruising this might have caused. It might be as well to mention that the Deputy was working his notice as he had taken a post with another authority. The Deputy had agreed to leave before the main party with the two boys to open the home and put the kettle on. While they were in the home and before the others returned a bunch of keys went missing including the keys to the safe. He asked the boys about the keys and they denied all knowledge. The Officer in Charge heard through the grapevine that this particular boy had really taken the keys and when the investigation had started he had thrown them away. Both boys were called into the office and confronted with the facts and placed on punishment. A short while later they absconded. Later the same day the Deputy saw them in town and gave chase. They led him to some derelict garages. The Deputy called the police who had been informed of the absconding and a policeman soon arrived in a Panda car. They also found a nineteen year old man there who was found to be an absconder from Borstal. The boys were taken back to the home by the Deputy. The next day they contacted the fieldworker and made their accusation.

A meeting was called two weeks later but just prior to this I asked the Officer in Charge of the Assessment Unit to which the boys were transferred what he had made of the boys. He said, "Trouble". The boy in question was the one who had cleaned a car with steel wool. It was obvious at the meeting that a lot of minds had been made up and that the deputy although not present, had been found guilty and this in spite of the fact that there was sketchy evidence from other children that the two boys were lying. The field staff wanted the boys returned to the home but the Officer in Charge was against this and pointed out that when the Deputy left, which would be quite soon, the boys would see themselves as having driven him out and this would consequently make the staff's position untenable, as anytime anything went wrong the same thing would happen again. Eventually I said I would not agree to either of the boys returning to the home and that the field worker would have to find an alternative place.

The sequel to this story is that boy in question went on to another home and later accused a member of staff of the same thing. He was moved on three occasions for the same reason and eventually he was sent to Borstal.

I had a story related to me about a man who was "drummed out" because a girl in the home had accused him of attempted rape. He admitted he was struggling with her because she had attacked him but he had to go.

Make no mistake staff are very vulnerable. Some may say that any man who attempts to deal with a girl alone is a fool. I would agree if there is female staff available but what does a man or woman do if they are alone on duty with a group of older children?

Many girls will goad male staff and even invite a man to strike them on the grounds that it could be sexual. Society and seniors think that where girls like this are concerned they must be right. Whichever way staff turn they are wrong. There is absolutely no understanding of what these types of children can be like. Some even prefer not to believe it.

Senior staff feel vulnerable but junior staff feel it even more. Seniors have some sanctions though weak ones, juniors have absolutely no authority. I have seen the strain such situations place upon a husband/wife team. Neither one would speak to the other the way the children speak to them. It is worse for the wife as, if she is being verbally abused or physically threatened the husband has to decide whether or not to interfere, because he is powerless and has to give his wife a chance to cope with the situation for her own good, as if he interferes it would be seen by some children as a lack of ability on the wife's part and would result in the wife facing some sort of confrontation at every turn. Such problems are always with the residential worker. They are not going home at 5 o'clock, they are more likely to be getting the same children up the next morning and short of leaving the work there is nothing staff can do about it. The intensity tears people apart and while field workers and residential staff are regarded as separate agencies there is no chance of anything positive being done in this work.

Some field workers regard a child they have taken into care as "their" child and will foolishly make the same mistake the child's parents have made, namely, defending them right or wrong and believing implicitly whatever the child says. I know of one field worker, when she heard that one of her clients had been arrested remark, "How dare they arrest one of my children, I'll soon sort them out."

There was a boy taken into care- his father was dead and he was beyond his mother's control. When he was allowed home he would extort money from his mother by threatening not to return unless he got it. Mother told the Officer in Charge and plans were made to stop it. Every time he returned from home any money was taken from him and a check made with his mother. His pocket money was monitored and if he bought anything his pocket money was checked. After a while staff began to feel pleased because they were making headway. Then one day they found he was getting money that they could not account for and all checks were negative. They were at a loss until out of the blue came the answer. One day staff found him showing money to other children having just been interviewed by the field worker. She had been bribing him to behave. Every time she saw him, she would ask if he had been a good boy and if as happened he said "Yes" he was rewarded with money. I do not propose to insult you by explaining what she was in fact doing but to coin a phrase "the mind boggles" and she had brought him into care![30]

Many children are recommended as being in need of a "structured environment" which in effect means a period of strict discipline and control, but where can one find such a place these days? At one time the approved schools or detention centres would provide this but not so in this enlightened age. Staff of children's homes get very bitter over the benefits of delinquents as opposed to non delinquents in care. If the delinquent happens to be in a normal children's home then staff can expect all sorts of excuses from reviews for any anti-social behaviour. If the child is affecting the other children adversely it will be said he/she will benefit from being with well behaved children. In fact what does happen more often than not is the reverse. The children soon realise that excuses are being made for bad behaviour and consequently they start on the same road and nothing staff say will make their seniors believe otherwise. Staff can tell the well behaved children this or that about Johnny being deprived or whatever, but as far as the children are concerned Johnny is simply getting away with it.

The children in homes will go to ordinary day school, 30 to 35 or more to a class. They will struggle with homework with others creating a racket around them. Many will do their best to behave, they will pay for themselves to go swimming or to the cinema and it is more than likely that the home will be an adapted property or a small house with limited play areas. However, if a child is sent to a community home school, as we call them now, it is more than likely there will be purpose built units with a quiet room, ideal for homework if they decide to do any. There will be 15 or so in a class. Special remedial teachers to coach them should they choose to take advantage of this. A private swimming pool is quite possible and a well equipped gymnasium maybe even a sports barn and certainly extensive playing fields. You think I am joking? I assure you that I am not. I worked in a school which was in the final stages if rebuilding. All that remained to be built when I left was a sports barn, swimming bath and an administration block. Staff children and their friends from the neighbourhood went to a school down the road which was 80 or 100 years old, classrooms made by sliding partitions across the room, 30/40 to a class, a small paved play area and the parents had to organise fund raising activities to buy books![31:32:33] I think society's priorities are wrong somewhere. Back to children in care. In the family group home the field worker will decide if the child can go home or not. In the community school the field worker will be told the school is closing and arrangements will have to be made for home leave. Often group homes have to make room for a child from a community school for a period of leave.

I know of one senior boys school where the headmaster made great play on the dignity of the boys and the home conditions they would return to. He ordered and received dressing gowns for all the boys. They were so used to this sort of life they showed them off as their nightshirts!

Field workers seem to be regarded as the professionals and residential workers as those who come after but have not quite reached the wonderful heights of professional status and many in the true professional style will tell the residential worker what they should do about a difficult child, and then leave or turn up with some bad news for the child but leave it to the residential worker to do the telling. The usual plea is, "Well you know him/her better than I, after all you are the residential worker and the one with the relationship"/ Not so at reviews, there you are only the residential worker not really worth listening to because it is then the field worker who has the relationship. The professionals decide, the non professionals perform. Let me say it is easy to tell someone what to do and run.

When society says a child is uncontrollable and should be in a home, then the residential worker is everything good, but let something happen and those same people will say how bad and wicked staff of homes are. Try telling a 17 year old to go to bed and he will tell you where to go or go out of a window and down the drainpipe. Smack him which might be a good thing and he will tell his mother and you can find yourself in Court facing an enquiry. Quite often staff cannot see any way of controlling an incident short of a smack, yet they dare not (that is unless they are prepared to take their career into their hands).

I have already mentioned the stress and frustrations generated in residential work and I would go so far as to say that it takes a very special type of person to do this work (any residential work) and survive, and it is time the people who order our lives developed the courage to take along hard look at the way things are going. Unfortunately it is the theorists who have the ear of policy makers and those who shape our lives in this work, yet it should be obvious even to the most ignorant that they are conspicuous by their absence in the homes.

There are a multitude of excuses for bad behaviour and we are bombarded with statistics as justification. When we are acquainted with the results of research into deviance and delinquency the theorists justify the results by saying "so much per cent had been proved, so we can assume the rest is correct" but this will only be said when it is in favour of their theories. When it is not in their favour we are told that the statistics are inconclusive. The theorists are, therefore, in a very strong position (heads I win, tails you lose). They will turn the world over to find some reason to excuse bad behaviour.

The following story should I hope serve to illustrate the point I have been trying to make.

I grew up close to a boy who went short of very little. We were all hard up in that neighbourhood but this boy's mother was a money lender, so he was never really short if a Saturday penny. He was better fed than most of us and unlike us he knew what holidays were. He started in a very small way stealing cigarettes, matches and small amounts of money from coats in parked vehicles. He always took another boy with him and when the police called it was always the other boy and never him. In fact, half the fathers in the street vowed what they would do to their children if they were to associate with this boy. His mother always supported him and told police what a good son he was and that it was the other children who were leading him astray. With his mother's help he escaped retribution for many years until he was eventually caught red handed and went down. There is no point in relating his career from then on sufficient to say he finished by doing fourteen years for armed robbery. He is dead now but from the stories which come back to me he got the sentence for planning and attempting a second great train robbery.

This boy was better off than most and no one could say his mother did not love him but she made the same mistake we are continually making today-refusing to believe that he was bad or naughty however you care to put it.

When we were young we were told that crime does not pay. The same cannot be said today. At the risk of repeating myself, children and adolescents are capable of thinking and arriving at conclusions. Have you ever stopped to think how many everyday things influence a child's thinking? For instance how many vehicles do you see obeying the speed limit in a built up area and when you read that someone has been caught what kind of sentences are handed out? A person can drive whilst drunk and kill someone. The result may well be an endorsement and a fine of £500. Children are quite capable of realising that this is the value society places on human life. On the other hand a person can be caught "fiddling" tax or social security benefits perhaps to the tune of several thousand pounds. The offender will be fined a few hundred pounds, usually these people finish up making a handsome profit. It has become quite a lucrative business for perpetrators of major crimes to write books about their criminal activities or for prominent people in public life to write their memoirs which usually include doubtful practices. Children see indifference at every turn. They see unions using "bully boy" tactics and encouraging people to do as little as possible for as much as they can get. They can also see frustrations of those trying to help them- particularly when battling against bureaucracy.

I had a group of boys all committed by the courts for offences. I had worked with them for a long time. In two years I had not had an absconding, bound breaking or court appearance. They had been very good with handicrafts and had made lots of articles to be sold at a fair. They would regularly take items home for sale to neighbours. They raised £170, all of it by their own efforts. We got to talking about holidays and I suggested a week or so on one of the islands off the West coast of Scotland, under canvas. They were very enthusiastic and I promised to start making arrangements and asked permission to take them. My request met with the reply, "It is not the policy of the authority to allow children to be taken out of the country." I said we would not require any money as we had enough of our own. It made no difference. I got the same reply. I pointed out that the Western Isles were part of Great Britain and still no use. This went on for weeks and all the time I was keeping the boys up to date. Eventually the boys and I had a meeting to discuss the situation. After a while one boy said, "It would be less bother if we all bunked it and met Mr Taylor in Scotland". He was perfectly right[37]. If you are going to look after children taken into care then you will have to be whiter than white because the children will take their lead from you. If you set low standards then that is all you can expect. Let us look at driving again. If you take a group of children out in a mini bus and exceed the limit then you are breaking the law and in effect are saying to all the children, "Its alright to break the law, as long as you don't get caught" or alternatively, if a person is in a position of influence or authority and breaks the law and gets away with it then children soon realise that it can be done and see no wrong in doing the same thing themselves. I have seen senior staff in some establishments blatantly stealing in one way or another and no matter how minor the incident may seem, it is still breaking the law.

I recall several incidents when I first entered residential work. I was with a boy one day when we witnessed one of these incidents. The boy said to me, "You know, Mr Taylor I was put in here for doing that". It was the most senior staff member who was involved and when the boy asked me why it was wrong for him but alright for others I was unable to give an honest answer.

One senior member of staff I worked with was an art teacher and he persuaded the committee to spend quite a sum of money to equip a room for craft purposes. His plea was that it would be therapeutic. He never took more than two boys one night a week, this out of one hundred boys. The rest of the time he used the equipment himself and replaced material out of school funds. He was on to a good thing and I often heard comments from boys on him and his activities. I can assure you that they were unprintable. I leave you to imagine how much benefit the boys gained from the therapy. Look around you and see just how many things influence the children you are trying to resocialise.[33:38]

I found in my dealings with children that a subtle approach is better than a blunt one, particularly if you have some sort of activity in mind. You do not have to be an expert in all things. If you are not sure of the activity but know how to start then tell the children and you can go on a voyage of discovery together. It pays to have "lots of strings to your bow" and it is fatal to say to a group of children, "Right we are going to do so and so, all sit down". I always had more success by taking something into my unit and working on it. The children's natural curiosity did the rest. Invariably they would gather round and ask questions and also if they could try. I found the same principle worked with adolescents as well.

You must also gear it to give them quick success otherwise you will fail. Gradually as they gain confidence and their tolerance threshold increases they will try the more difficult things. Think carefully about anything you intend starting for if you have any sense you should have a reason other than entertainment, though to the onlooker or the children it may well have to appear purely entertaining.

Let me give you an example.

I have always had a lot of hobbies and I will try anything in the craft line. One I am quite fond of is marquetry and this involves using very sharp craft knives and I thought long and hard about starting it. I had some very aggressive boys and I was looking for a constructive way of reducing their aggression (kicking one another whilst playing soccer only exacerbated it- something which also affects children when they see it on television). However I decided to try so I took some veneers and glue etc. into the unit one evening and started. It was only a matter of minutes before half a dozen boys were sitting with me asking questions and wanting to try. I had prepared my ground well beforehand. I had several simple pictures and had gathered together enough materials to start a dozen boys but they had to wait a couple of nights before they got properly started. There were certain conditions imposed, e.g. they had to use their own glue, if they broke a knife blade they had to pay for a replacement and they had to use a cutting board. Their motor co-ordination was poor to start with but it soon improved and they were not long in tackling some quite complicated pictures and were very proud of the finished articles. It was also noticeable that the incidence of aggression dropped. A problem arose which I had not foreseen. One boy who had an I.Q. of 56 could not get the hang of it and he was wasting a lot of veneers and rapidly losing heart. I pounded my brain to find a solution then it came to me. I went to a wallpaper printing firm and begged from them several rolls of waste wallpaper with simulated wood veneer patterns. I gave them to this boy with a pair of scissors. It was a success and he was able to make pictures just like the others and was perfectly happy doing it. I never forced boys to carry on once they had started. If anyone wanted to put it away it was alright with me. Over a period of time I introduced half a dozen or so activities using the same ploy. Stone polishing was introduced by them seeing me trying to polish a pebble with a piece of wet and dry emery paper. From there it was a small step to making jewellery. Hornwork started by my working on a boat made out of cow's horn. I must have been doing something right for I have seen my unit built to accommodate fifteen boys, with forty boys all working happily away and no one forced them to come- they chose to.[33]

You may think to yourself that is all very well but where did the money come from. The short answer is- from the boys themselves. I put it to them if they each subscribed three pence a week from their pocket money we would buy materials, make articles and sell them. The profits we would plough back until the activities became self financing. I used to hold a meeting with them once a month when they would get a simple balance sheet and also decide what materials needed replacing and what new ideas they wanted to try. My wife still has a necklace made for her by one of the boys.

Now for all this I was disciplinarian. If a boy broke the rules inside school or the law outside then he was in for punishment of some sort and they knew it. If a boy committed a crime while he was with me and I was sure in my own mind he had then he got no protection from me. In fact I would inform the police. If, on the other hand, I felt sure the boy had not done what he was accused of then he could count on me for help. They all knew if I caught them lying to me just once I would never believe them again. I will tell you now that you can be as strict as you wish with children providing you are honest, fair and just. In spite of what the so-called experts say, children need clear guidelines. They need to know how far they can go. Do not waste your time trying to fool children for, as I have already said, they have assessed you for what you are long before you ever get round to them. I have had my failures and I admit it. Alright I have read the books written by the Gurus of Child Care who only ever declare success and then wait for the faithful to worship at their feet and pick up any pearls of wisdom they choose to drop. These people are afraid. Afraid to say "I don't know." They are afraid because they think such an admission reflects adversely upon their ability. in fact it takes an honest person to admit they are not the fountain of knowledge and it is some other poor residential worker who suffers through their stupidity since by the time they have finished playing about with a problem child the time has passed when any good can be done.[43]

If you need to punish a child or young person it should be done there and then. None of this "Wait until your father gets home" attitude or "I'll tell the Officer in Charge because all you are doing is making someone out to be the ogre. I have had children caned. I would have done it myself but only the Head or Deputy was allowed to do so. I have also recommended the cane in assessment reports and am not ashamed to admit it. I recall one boy I had caned after he had been abusive and he changed for the better within a week. In fact to my knowledge he did not get into trouble with the police again. When he left me he got a job and the last we heard he was doing very well. If ever you have to punish, do it and then forget it. Do not rake it up again. One thing which infuriates me is seeing the group punished for the misdemeanours of one. Usually because the staff do not have the courage to deal with the situation themselves. The thought behind this is the group will do my job for me and punish the wrongdoer. This only encourages bullying, then the children are punished for doing that. Obviously there are grey areas. If a brick came through the window smashing the glass and you caught four children then they should all share the cost, providing the culprit did not own up but to use the group to enforce discipline is wrong and unjust. Often and I repeat, often, with the right kind of relationships you will find out who the wrongdoers are. If you want to establish trust and maintain discipline you will have to put yourself out to a considerable degree and you will have to think carefully about what you are going to do and how you are going to do it. Never make a promise if you cannot fulfil it and never threaten anything unless you can carry it out. I have heard staff threaten "fire and brimstone" knowing full well they would not be able to do it. The only thing this will earn you is contempt and once you have shown you cannot carry out your threat you will have lost credibility in the eyes of the children. Field workers and staff of homes make promises without thinking. Understand this. Children will take out of a conversation only what suits them and when the promise is not fulfilled the child or children react and some poor staff member will be in the line of fire, so, put your brain into gear before you put your tongue into motion. In short THINK. Children may well lie to you but they expect the absolute truth from you. If you do lie to children and they find out it is highly unlikely they will trust your word again. If you suspect that a child is lying to you, you will be very foolish if you just accept it as one of those things that all children do these days. Check what is said even if it means putting yourself to some trouble, eventually you will find out the truth and form a better relationship.

Residential workers, if they are doing their job, have to be awake to everything in the home. Get the little things right and the big things will be easier. Once they realise that you are going to see that they wash, clean their teeth or polish their shoes properly they will also realise that you are awake to the big things. Intervening in situations at the right time, before it gets to the punishment stage, be aware of what is play and what is in earnest. There are so many signs which you must learn to interpret, these are just some of the skills the residential worker must develop. I know some people will skoff at this, but good residential workers develop a sixth sense. One worker with that sense is worth five without. A good worker can step into a group and know when there is something wrong. The same with individuals, the worker will know the behaviour pattern so well he will detect the slightest variation.

The biggest boost to my ego was given unwittingly by one of the worst little tearaways I ever handled. I asked him to look after a new boy. When he got around the corner of the building and imagined he was out of earshot he said, "That's Mr. Taylor he doesn't miss a trick so don't try being smart with him". I felt I had arrived.

Many people in social work talk very glibly about relationships after a few days. Worthwhile relationships take time and patience. If you imagine you have a meaningful relationship with a child after a few days, just because of the child's friendly attitude towards you, then you are being very childish. He is more likely to be probing your defences. Some staff, both residential and fieldwork, lose heart because the relationships they want to fail to materialise.

Their next move is usually to give everything they can in order to get the children on their side. This is nothing less than bribery. They may buy conformity for a while but it certainly will not last.

Residential work with Children - Balbernie

The work has to be professionally disciplined. Staff are there to deal skilfully with the fact of separation, emotional deprivation, parental malfunction; for in these gaps and spaces in experience and in the actual suffering and disturbance they cause lies also the possibility for healing through increased consciousness. These wounds and weaknesses are themselves the agents for health; if this can be realised, then through them things can take a very different turn. In unskilled hands this opportunity for healing is lost for the staff may then blindly fall into quasi- parental, possessive (mothering or fathering) roles, attempting to fill in the gaps, or may attempt to minister to these wounds by covering them up with cotton wool and bandages- responses which reflect only their own unconscious emotional needs.

24. Peters, writing on moral education underlines this:

    For moral education is a matter of initiating others into traditions and into procedures for revising and applying them; these come to be taken in as habits of mind. It is also a matter of spreading the contagion of sympathy and imagination so that such traditions bite on behaviour. But I think we have little established knowledge about the crucial conditions which favour the initiation into this distinctive form of life.

25. That the regime should be democratic and non-punitive, though structure, control, authority and security are likely to be critical considerations. Adult roles need to be active, participant and responsive, sensitive following of mutually created roles in therapeutic involvement. No single imposed pattern of leadership is required.

    It should reflect the qualities of a really good family and home, but in fact, be much more than and essentially other than this in a much more deliberate and conscious offering of additional relationship security, unconditional acceptance, and specific remedial and corrective treatment. The family concept only causes task confusion. Every child has two parents.

37. Pretence, omnipotence, and unreality beget omnipotence, unreality and activate fantasies, which interrupt communication about real things at all levels, and special experience and consciousness in leadership in groups is required in this field and in the maintenance of the healing climate of a therapeutic community. The dead hand of unconscious bureaucracy welcomes the collusive off-loading and distribution of responsibility into the functionally autonomous powerishness, and omnipotence which develops in committees.

38. Special educational opportunities. Intellectual stimulation. Sense of achievement, competence, and worth in performance of skills. Gratification in their performance modifying the need for immediate impulsive instinctual gratifications. Opportunity for continuous sense of achievement. Skilled vocational guidance, assessment, and preparation.

Residential Life with Children- C. Beedell

31. Research findings over the past thirty years have moved to the conclusion that the capacity for intelligent behaviour can in large measure be acquired. This being so the educative function of residential units become more important and the intellectual capacities of those staffing them need to be as high as possible if children in them, albeit damage or deprive, are not to be given second-class opportunities of development.

32. Physical provision. Problems of finance, staffing ratios, etc., have already been mentioned. Two particular problems have received insufficient attention in the past; space and buildings. The amount and kind of space required in residential units has not received much study. This is partly for reasons of economy, partly because we have not re-thought traditional block provision for those with special needs. The amount of space which should be available for a child in his own house has already been mentioned in relation to play.

Child Care and the Growth of Love- J. Bowlby

23. In all countries there is much debate in medical circles regarding treatment given by non-medical workers, but, though they still have their critics; it is safe to say they have come to stay. Those psychiatrists who have actually had experience of working with social workers and psychologists in this way are almost unanimous regarding their value, though they would emphasise the need for them to be properly trained and to work in close collaboration with a doctor trained and experienced in psychological treatment.

27. Until more effective measures for restoring health to psychologically ill characters can be found, or until long term measures of mental hygiene have proved successful in preventing their development, this indeed may be the right solution.

30. The parent is held to the need to examine the nature of the neglect, to determine what he can do about it, to explore whether that will help meet the child's needs, and to recognize how the agency stands ready to help him achieve for the child the needed care and security...(he) must be helped to know the limitations as well as the advantages of boarding care as the case worker knows them.

    Here perhaps, is the crux of the matter-'as the case worker knows them'. So long as the case workers do not know these limitations, but live, as some do, in the sentimental glamour of saving neglected children from wicked parents, they will act impetuously in relieving parents of their responsibilities and, by their action, convey to the parents the belief that the child is far better off in the care of others. Only if the case worker is mature enough and trained enough to respect even bad parents and to balance the less evident long term considerations against the manifest and perhaps urgent short term ones, will she help the parents themselves and do a good turn to the child.

33. Arising out of this field of animal research, however, a number of psychologists have been led to suggest that the key factor in 'maternal deprivation' is in reality not the lack of relationship with a mother

figure but something quite different, namely inadequate stimulation from the environment. This has led Yarrow, in a recent review of the literature on maternal deprivation, to emphasize the need for research to analyse the deprivation experience into its components of sensory, social and emotional deprivation.

While we agree that further research of this nature is highly desirable, and while we agree that, in comparison with the average family environment, an institution environment is often monotonous, barren in emotional tone and meagre in environmental stimulation.

The special question of delinquency. Particular controversy has centred upon delinquency as an outcome of maternal deprivation. Bender applied the term 'psychopathic behaviour disorder' to the clinical syndrome she found associated with early and severe deprivation experiences. An early study of Bowlby's used juvenile thieves as subjects, and demonstrated an association between the 'affectionless character' shown by some of the most persistent of them and early, severely depriving separation experiences.

Bowlby suggested that experiences of this nature may be foremost among the causes of 'delinquent character formation'. These and similar findings and opinions of other early investigations, have led to the widely held belief that the hypothesis that maternal deprivation causes later maladjustment or disorder necessarily implies that deprivation always or frequently causes delinquency. As it turns out, delinquency had not been found to be a common outcome of maternal deprivation or early mother child separation; and this has led some critics to conclude that deprivation itself is not damaging.

The relationship between early separation and/or deprivation experiences and delinquency remains controversial because evidence derived from different sorts of research appears to conflict. Evidence derived from retrospective case studies of psychiatrically disturbed children and adults regularly demonstrates a significant association between, on the one hand, behaviour disorder and character disorders including 'affectionless' character and, on the other, severe, early, and depriving separation experience. Thus one study of children in a guidance clinic shows that conduct disorders, including stealing, occur significantly more frequently among children from homes broken by the loss of one parent through death, divorce, or separation than among children from intact homes. When they do occur among children from intact homes, moreover, conduct disorders are more frequent in those who have been separated from their mothers than in other children.

Exceptional Children – Lenhoff

28. The role of the visiting psychiatrist to Shotton Hall deserves special mention here. In many ways he serves as a go-between for staff and children. With his specialized knowledge of diagnosis and prognosis, he can often give timely warnings of dangers of which we should be on the lookout in certain cases, e.g. likely explosive acts, or depressions and regressions. He can also give tips towards beneficial treatment, because he often has more intimate details about a case then we have, as a result of confidence given by the child, just because he can see things more in perspective, being less involved than we are personally in the outcome of a boy's stay at our school.

29. Whatever the main motive of a school's work, each has something special to give to a particular kind of child, and this the psychiatrist and his team can judge best after consultation wit the school.

Residential Work with Children – R. Balbernie

Environmental control. Opportunity for environment control, specially planned opportunity for self government and for participation in community organizations (i.e. courts) and for social learning. Within the opportunity for individuality, the opportunity for sharing in responsibility (shared individual responsibility; this is quite a different state from shared irresponsibility which is motivated, collusive and projective distribution of responsibility). This requires skilled group psychotherapy in which the leader is especially conscious of tendencies to project (and evade) individual responsibility in to the 'we' or outwards into 'them' or upwards to hierarchical leadership.

Residential Care Reviewed P.S.S.C.1977

75. We have been made aware in our work that many staff feel unsupported. It is obvious that some of the systems that are in existence for providing support do not function as well as they should, and it can be very easy for those managing the systems to be unaware of how staff in their homes feel. Attention should be paid therefore, not only to the setting up of support systems where they do not exist, but also to examining those that do exist, to see if they do, in fact, give to staff the encouragement and sense of confidence that is intended.

Gurus

43. While I was on a placement in a well known community school I talked to one of the senior staff about child care and the conversation got around to the books which at that time were being used as 'Bibles' on the courses.

The name of one person, an author of several books, was mentioned. This man was considered by my tutors and many of the colleagues on the course to be the leading light in the Child Care Field, anything written by him was avidly read, his success, from his writing was considered by us to be phenomenal and was held up to us as something we should aim for as he never seemed to have a failure. Students queued to get placements with him.

I was told by a member of staff that failure would never be mentioned by this man because on paper he didn't have any. He went on to explain how he and others in the school had discovered what actually was happening. If a child was considered to be in need of a placement in this great man's establishment the usual request would be made and copies of the case history obtained. It might be anything up to three months before they heard anything. if the child was considered as a suitable admission there would be an interview for the child with the great man (this would reduce the risk of failure to start with)and on this basis there would be acceptance or rejection.

The member of staff said he and others often saw faces they knew among children and when they had checked up they had found that these children were among rejects from the great man's establishment. Having admitted them and found he could do nothing for them they were quietly slipped back into the mainstream of admissions to the school and consequently never showed as failures – it was as if they had never been there. This man due to his success had the ear of policy makers and has exercised considerable influence on the child care field.

As I have already said he is king of the country of the blind who has one eye.

Chapter 6

We are regularly acquainted with the findings of research into residential care (not just children). Usually a sample number is quoted and the inference behind the theories is, if you do this or that, in a given set of circumstances then the problem will be solved. One thing they all seem to forget (including course tutors) is, all things are not the same to all men. The human being is about the most complicated animal on the face of the earth. You can embark on a course of action with one person/ child because of a disturbance or problem and achieve success. You can use the same course of action for the same problems on a different person and fail completely.

I learned a very bitter lesson with a boy once. He was committed by the court for a string of offences over a period of time. His fieldworker brought him and admitted he was at the end of his tether with the boy. He was with me for eighteen months. From the first week he displayed a willingness to make an effort. He went to school regularly, did his work and showed consistent improvement. He stayed away from the trouble makers when he was on leave. All the staff and his fieldworker were extremely pleased with his progress. His parents came to see me and said what a change we had made in him. It was inevitable in view of his behaviour that a case conference be convened and the consensus of opinion was that he should be sent home. To be on the safe side we decided to defer sending him home until after we had "tapped the grapevine" just to see if the rest of the children could come up with anything we had missed. We could find nothing to make us change or minds and so he was sent home. Within two weeks his fieldworker was in contact. The boy was as bad as ever. He was stealing, hanging around with gangs and sleeping in derelict property. His parents were in despair. He had fooled everyone, staff, teachers, fieldworker and children. He went on to an Intermediate Approved

School. It taught me a lesson I have tried not to forget.

It is reasonable to assume that if you are in residential work for any length of time you get a child who is potentially more intelligent than you are. I am referring to a child with a high I.Q. I admit if this happens you will be taxed to the limit. If you are not awake to your job this child will run rings round you. I have seen children like this labelled as maladjusted mainly because people who had dealt with the child before you, have felt affronted at the realisation that they were the intellectual inferior of a child. The child is often looked upon as a "know all" or "show off" or just a nuisance. It is a strange thing that adults refuse to face the fact that a child can be very intelligent and will go to great lengths to suppress any sign or move the child on to some one else- anything as long as they are not faced with the constant remainder that they are expected to cater for this type of child. It may well be that the child has criminal tendencies, if so admit they are highly intelligent and that they have such tendencies. It does not do the child or society any good if you label them with some obscure mental [40] disturbance just because you feel personally offended. If you do get such a child who is criminally inclined they will very likely play havoc with the group and you will need all your wits about you to maintain any sort of stability as children will take more notice of their peers than they will of you. I know there is nothing worse than seeing perhaps years of patient work being destroyed after the admission of a child like this and the mental smarting when they smile at you while their eyes say, " I've beaten you and you can't do a thing about it". Alternatively you could get high I.Q. child who is in need of mental stimulation. This can also present problems. They have no criminal inclinations at all but they will still tax you.

I have found in cases like this where you are unable to cater for them it helps them and you to find someone who can, or encourage the child to do it themselves.

I had a boy with an I.Q. of 142, even the other boys called him "professor". I was worried about him because he was slowly moving towards the criminal element in the unit and I realised that if he finally established himself there I would have real trouble. I had a somewhat tenuous relationship with him as he was never very forthcoming. I have found this with many high I.Q. children. I managed, however, to get him in a talkative mood and I did it over a game of draughts. It came out that he was interested in electronics and found pleasure in trying to repair transistor radios. His school work reports left a lot to be desired, particularly his mathematics. He was obviously following the same pattern as his peers. I had a talk with one of his teachers who worked very closely with me and we always kept one another informed about what was happening with the children. It was agreed what course of action we would take. I would sow the seeds in the unit and he would develop it in the classroom. I allowed the boy to bring in transistors which he wanted to repair and in fact found a couple for him. I started my moves by asking him how they worked, 'He was most expansive in his explanations and this gave me the opportunity I needed. I hinted to him that electronic engimers relied very heavily on formal education particularly mathematics. It was not long before his teacher said he was begining to ask questions. The teacher had to play things very carefully and had to relate what he was doing to the boy's interest and the boy had to see some results for his efforts. During my talks with him, - I found that although he had been committed by the court for breaking telephones, he had never taken any money — all he wanted was the instrument which he would take to pieces and use the parts to build calculators, admittedly they were very "Heath Robinson" and had their limitations. He brought one he had built to show me and I admit I was very impressed. The improvement in the boy's behaviour and attitude was slow at first but soon gathered momentum and it was not too long before his school reports stated that he was like a sponge where learning was concerned. I am not sure whether I should count this boy's progress as a success as he left school and got himself into trouble - not with the police this time with a girl. I will not go into more details as be will be a man now with a family of his own.

There is no distinction these days between good and bad. As I have said where now can we find establishments where discipline will be imposed. Family group homes are now expected to fulfill this role and are often condemned for doing it. If you have a settled group of children and can watch the results of your efforts it is very satisfying but get one delinquent placed amongst them and it is not long before people in the neighborhood begin to refer to all the children as "those little horrors from that home". They all get labelled.

Many children come into care through no fault of their own, neglected, abandoned, orphaned and they have not been in trouble with the police. To expose them to criminal or delinquent influences is, in my opinion, criminal in itself, yet try getting this influence removed and you find yourself up against a stone wall. You will be asked or told to make allowances and you will continue to be asked to make allowances until the child goes to a detention centre or Borstal then it will be intimated that you have failed in your Job. Children may be considered to be in moral danger and brought into care and may well be in more danger in care. I have already quoted an example.

A lot of people with questionable motives gravitate towards work with children, which increases their vulnerability. Look around you, the law of permissiveness has now become license. Having found such people getting them out is nearly impossible - have you tried doing it lately? When such staff hit the headlines residential care is condemned and all staff of homes are monsters, no mention is made of the hundreds of staff who work quietly and devotedly against all the odds for the benefit of their charges.

The latest band wagon is a children's charter. It will be interesting to see what it contains. I admit that children have rights but then, so do staff and the public in general. The people who establish these rights have got it wrong for the last thirty years and all I have to say to them is "Don't get it wrong for the next thirty'. There will be a lot of people climbing on this bandwagon but the last to be consulted will be those at the grass roots. They are the ones who have to make it work.

There is a group of people set up by the D.H.S.S. They have for a while now been gathering children in care into groups to discuss their feelings and views on residential care. I have been to a preliminary meeting held by these people, one admitted quite openly that they knew nothing at all about residential work, yet it would appear from some of the stories I have heard that they have everything to do with the Charter so it would appear quite possible that the residential worker will again be told how the job should be done by people who know nothing at all about it.

I accept some of the complaints children have about their care but I do not accept complaints by those who break the law and abuse staff.. I am the first to agree that children have the right to a say in their future, there is nothing new in these ideas sensible residential workers have been discussing with children future plans for some time now. I remember one idea that children should have some say in punishment. I wonder would those who float these ideas act on the children's wishes? I had a boy who was caught stealing from the others. We had a meeting about it and the opinion of the children was, "Chop his bloody hands off!" Residential workers were told they must not use any form of coercion to maintain discipline yet delinquent types use coercion in many bizarre ways to enforce their will upon the individual. One constantly reads reports of the misery some children suffer in school through bullying, even to the point of setting fire to any child considered to have transgressed, even handicapped children have no immunity from young thugs and parents in this culture will refute any accusations against their children and make no effort to discipline them. Let children do their own thing! One type I was always very hard on was the bully and it was also one of the few things my headmaster would cane for.

Society is wrong! So we are told by a section of the self same society. Get rid of the slum properties, provide more facilities for youngsters, give, give, give, having done all that the problems will be solved. To a great extent this has been done and the standard of living in this country has never been higher yet the juvenile crime rate is breaking all records.

Liverpool Council thought they had taken giant strides towards solving the problem yet some years ago they built a whole new housing estate then moved the slum dwellers out to their new houses and pulled down the old property. The city fathers have had to admit it has not worked. The estate is now a modern slum. At the risk of sounding facetious even the police dogs walk round in pairs.[41]

Before closing the section on children I would like to relate several cases all of which have some effect on residential workers. They all happened in the same authority and staff who were involved were very bitter and I must confess to being defeated by the logic. There was a senior housemother whose husband had left her with five children. She lived in a small three bedroom terraced house, and worked hard to bring her children up properly. They were a credit to her, went to school regularly, studied hard, never knocked around in gangs and. were never in trouble. The housemother paid her rent and bills regularly and owed nothing to anyone. As her children were growing up she asked the local authority for a four bed roomed house. The Housing Department were very polite but sorry there was no chance. In the same terrace of houses there was another woman whose children had been taken into care several times. She paid no one and gas and electricity had been cut off. The housemother was astounded when the woman was given a four bed roomed house which was furnished for her and included a coloured television and a telephone. All outstanding debts were settled.

Five children were found in a house, the oldest being seven and the youngest fifteen months. They were taken into care overnight.. The next morning the mother turned up and demanded her children. She said she and her husband wanted a night out. She got her children and nothing was said or done.

I only hope the children's charter includes some protection for children whose parents treat them like this.

One Officer in Charge got a call from a fieldworker asking for a food parcel for four people. This was on Friday night. After getting permission from his senior the Officer in Charge made up a big parcel of food. On Monday the full story was obtained from the fieldworker. The four people, a woman, her cohabitee, her son –and a young woman lodger had gone to a night club and spent the money which had been given to them by the Social Security department. They had also lost their social security card in the night club. Having had a night out and spent all their money they phoned the duty officer.

People like those in the cases above are not inadequate – they just do not care.

Now compare the last two cases with the following:

A seventeen and a half year old girl due to go out of care was told if she could find suitable accommodation she could leave whenever she wished. She was a good girl, went to work regularly and saved what she could out of a modest wage, having paid for her keep in the hostel. Moves where made to help her get a flat from the Housing Department. Eventually she had a flat in a suitable area. She calculated she could just pay the rent if she could get some help with furnishings. She was told that the social services as good parents would help. Everything she thought would be alright. Finally the time came to move and she got her financial help - £25. She could not buy a decent coat for that price these days. She could not afford to furnish and pay the rent, so had to move to a bed sitting room in a not so suitable area. As it happened the girl kept her dignity and self respect yet had she turned to anti-social behaviour the local authority would have said "After all we did for her".[42]

These days it does not pay to try and make an honest effort on your own behalf. Get into trouble and all the considerable machinery of social services, D.H.S.S. and society security moves into action on your behalf and excuses will be made for the predicaments you get yourself into. Make a genuine effort and nobody wants to know.

Residential Work with Children – R. Balbernie

40. Reid and Hagan wrote in 1952 of conditions in the States and of off loading residual and labelled populations:

They have been established to provide treatment for the child for whom Child Guidance Clinics, foster care agencies, family agencies, and corrective institutions have been unable to provide adequate help. They have been described as incorrigible, untreatable; have been ousted from public schools and rejected by neighborhood and community. Many of these cases have so baffled the ordinary attempt of psychiatric treatment that their diagnoses have been relegated to the catch - all nosological wastepaper basket. They are labelled with obscure and non - verifiable defects such as constitutional psychopaths.

41. The proper care of children deprived of a normal home life can now be seen to be not merely an act of common humanity, but to be essential for the mental and social welfare of a community. For, when their care is neglected, as still happens in every country of the Western World today, they grow up to reproduce themselves. Deprived children, whether in their own homes or out of them, are the source of social infection as real and serious as are carriers of diphtheria and typhoid. And, just as preventive measures have reduced these diseases to negligible proportions, so can determined action greatly reduce the number of deprived children in our midst and the growth of adults likely to produce more of them. An economic system which from time to time creates unrelieved poverty on a scale so great that social workers are powerless to help.

Consolidation of child care legislations – Howard Bishop
Social work today vol. II N°. 33 29.4.80

42. Duty of local authorities to promote welfare of children. Section I of the 1963 Act has been superseded by Section I of the 1980 Act, whereby it is the <u>duty</u> of every local authority to make available such advice, guidance and assistance as may promote the welfare of children by diminishing the need to receive children into, or keep them in care,

including provision for giving assistance in kind, or in <u>exceptional</u> <u>circumstances in cash.</u>

Chapter 7

Although this book is about Residential Work and Residential workers views some who read it may be inclined to say, "That is all very well but we are not in a position to answer back" so to this end I approached a Field worker and asked if he would like to comment. The person I approached enjoys a great deal or respect from all residential staff he comes into contact with. The following is a record of the conversation he and I had.

Q. We often hear a lot about the gulf that exists between Field and Residential staff. What are your feelings about this?

A. I feel that once I put a child into a home the residential staff and I must work together. I don't expect them to be at me all the time. Can I do this or can I do that? I do expect them to keep me informed.

Q. That means that you are prepared to give residential staff autonomy to deal with a child as they think right within a set agreement between them and you?

A. Yes. If staff say to me can Johnny go home this weekend I usually ask if he deserves to go home. If the answer is Yes then I will agree, see the parents and if they agree then its fine with me. I think this is the sort of situation which can break relationships. I don't say no a child can't go home, I rely on the judgement of the residential staff.

Q. Can we develop that a bit more? A lot of field workers will go to the residential staff and say, "I say that such a body can't do this, that or the other" then walk away and leave it to the residential worker to tell the child and face the back lash when the child says, "Its you who won't let me do it" when in point of fact it is the field worker. How do you feel about this?

A. I feel that it is up to the field worker to tell a child what he or she has decided not leave it to the staff in the home. This is just foisting responsibility onto others. Say the Field worker decides a child should not go home, it is then up to him to go to his client and say why he has made such a decision. He should make it quite plain to the child that it is he and not the residential worker who will not let him go home. I feel this helps greatly in cementing relationships between residential and field staff. With this approach I can work on a child and know we are working to the same end. I expect to be kept fully in the picture, if say a child was doing wrong or getting into trouble then if the staff need my support they only need to ask and I will go to the home and see the child.

Q. Following on what you have just said how do you feel about colleagues of yours who get a call from home and say, "Don't bother me do such and such. I have other things to do"

A. They are shirking their responsibilities. I maintain that if they have a child in a home it is just as though they had their own child in their own home. It is up to the field worker to see that their client is being cared for and if the child is complaining about a home it is up to him to see the residential staff and sort out the problem.

Q. Case conferences too often become a clash of wills between the residential and field worker. How do you think we can get over this sort of thing?

A. If both think they are right why not give both ideas a chance over an agreed period of time.

Q. Do you think this clash of wills often happens?

A. Yes! Very often. Sometimes the field worker thinks a decision isn't right and the residential worker thinks it is then there is bound to be a conflict but lets face it, we get conflict in our own homes with our own children.

Q. Yes but what I'm getting at is, do you think it happens on many occasions because when I was in residential work I never had a bad relationship with any of my field workers. I have often felt annoyed about a decision but have gone ahead with it and if it didn't prove right I've gone the other way and I've told the field worker "This way isn't producing the results we want, now I'm going to try something else". I continually get complaints from residential staff who say this doesn't happen and that one course of action is imposed on them and on occasions the decision of the case conference is over ruled by someone higher up. How do you feel about this?

A. You mean been over ruled by the hierarchy. This is like the field worker over ruling the residential worker. I think this is wrong, after all it is myself and the residential staff who are dealing with the client.

Q. Can we develop this a bit further? In a case conference you can have anything up to ten people present and as you no doubt know the more people you have trying to make a decision the less likely you are to get one. Do you feel (and this is an idea of my own which I used to practice) that all information is fed into the case conference but the ultimate decision is between the field and residential worker and not to try to reach a collective decision.

A. I feel that at a case conference more attention should be paid to residential staff comments. After all the child is living in that home, the staff know the child's faults and attitudes and the report they make should be taken very seriously. It is all very well for people like me or members of the hierarchy to turn up to a conference when we may only see a child for half an hour a week, if that. The residential worker is living with that child twenty four hours a day and their views must be taken into consideration.

Q. Can we talk about punishment? Corporal punishment, mental punishment, etc. What are your views on this?

A. We are supposed to be a progressive society. There is a lot of talk about bringing back the birch but if you asked me to give the birch I would have to say no. I couldn't hurt a child by birching so I have no right to ask for its restoration. There we have to say, "What is the next best thing?" I admit with my own children I have had the occasion to smack and I feel it hasn't done them any harm. I've always been sorry after I have done it and questioned my own motives.

Q. Yes. What concerns me as a residential worker is the fact that I have seen a child nearly destroyed by bad staff using mental punishment. I would sooner have seen that child get a clip across the ear and forget it. This is what I am trying to get at. A member of staff says, "Right, I can't smack so I will screw that child down so tight he will be useless to anyone afterwards and no marks will show." Which would you prefer of the two?

A. I would prefer the corporal punishment. I think that once we start using that form of punishment we have lost a child. If we set out to reduce a child to a mental wreck we have lost them for good. But if we smacked we would lose them for a short time and then they would come back.

Q. So many of your colleagues say that corporal punishment is out. Alright it is accepted in residential care that you are not supposed to use it and as I say so many of your colleagues feel this way that there are now no sanctions other than mental manipulation which can be brought to bear and this distresses me greatly.

A. I must say this. Just over a month ago one of the homes sent for me because one of the children was refusing to go to school and they could do nothing to make him. I'm afraid I gave him a rough time and he went to school. I took him in the car and on the way I stopped and had a long talk with him and pointed out that the home staff were concerned about his future. I also told him that if ever he wanted to talk to me he was to ask the staff to get me on the telephone. That very same night he took me at my word and rang me. Alright I used the strong arm method but I feel it strengthened our relationship in this case and the boy is only about nine.

Q. If you have thought it necessary would you have gone further?

A. I wouldn't like to answer that one. I think it depends on what circumstances a person finds themselves faced with. I prefer to deal with staff in small homes than in assessment centres, although they are supposed to be better educated.

Q. Do you mean better educated or consider themselves more expert?

A. Well. Consider themselves to be more expert. I have on two occasions had good reason to mistrust their judgement. One, I had a boy who had been to a school for the maladjusted and to a couple of community schools, detention centres three times and a remand home. It was decided here that he should be reassessed. He was a real headache. Among other things he had stolen nine cars and crashed two of them so it was decided to send him back to a well known assessment centre to be reassessed. To me, our department wasted their money because the assessment was that he should be allowed to go back home. I questioned this and asked if I brought another boy of the same type would they suggest sending him. I told them he could steal another car and possibly kill someone. They said, "Well if he does that you can send him to Borstal". I could have sent him to Borstal but I wanted some positive help and suggestions with this boy. Anyway he went home and within a matter of weeks he stole another car and went to Borstal. He is still there.

Another case I had a boy in the cells and went to collect him. People may think I am cruel but I took him to the car in his stocking feet with his trouser fly open. People asked why and I told them that he couldn't run that way. I hadn't had him out of the cells more than a minute when he tried to break. We managed to get him into the car and for about three miles I was trying to drive and fight him. As luck would have it there was a police car behind me so I stopped them and asked for help. One of them came with me and we took him to an assessment centre. I won't mention the name. We had to handcuff this lad, he was a real hard case, sixteen years old with the body of a man. When we got to the assessment centre the first words from the superintendent were, "Take those handcuffs off the boy. I don't allow that sort of thing here". I took the handcuffs off and he said "Thank you goodbye." We got back into the car and I apologized to the policeman for the superintendent's attitude and said I hoped the boy ran away that night, and as it happened he did. That boy is now in Borstal. These people are supposed to be dealing with boys of this kind and they are suppose to be highly educated yet they behave to the police and field workers in this way so what chance has a child got?

I can see your dilemma. Having been in charge of an assessment unit I feel that until you have had a chance to come to some conclusions about a new admission you should not make valued judgements and until such time you must take the field workers views into consideration. I feel that in assessment it should be an even closer liasion with the field worker because if at the end of the assessment period it is decided that no positive suggestions or course of action can be offered then the field worker has the nasty job of trying to find a suitable placement.

Q. Are you in favour of senior staff in assessment units talking to a child's parents in their home? I used to but so many of your colleagues object to this.

A. I'm all in favour of it. Particularly if it will help the child. I knew a superintendent of an assessment centre who would take the child home for a day and see what conditions were for himself. I have recently taken over a case of a maladjusted boy who is in an assessment centre. The superintendent of the centre has moved house to this town. I telephoned him and offered to show him around. I took him to a couple of our homes and then took him to see where the boy lived and I think it opened his eyes to see what the boy was going back to.

Q. Do you think it will help the assessment?

A. Most certainly. We had a meeting about it the other week and it has been decided to keep him at the centre until he gets a job because to send him back to those conditions to kick his heels day after day would end in disaster for him and I feel that this has done the boy a power of good.

Q. How do you fell about bribing children to get them into a home? So often when I was in residential work I found that children had been bribed with cigarettes, sweets or money just to get them to the door of the home without any trouble or the fact that the field worker hadn't told them they were going into a home until they got them to the door and leaving the residential worker to face the problems.

A. Any field worker that does that sort of thing should be sacked. Once you start bribing a child you are admitting you are beaten and also it opens too many doors to a child to know right away they can manipulate you. This should never be, if a child is going into a home it is the field worker's duty to tell him and not just leave him at the door but take him in and introduce him and make sure he is settled before leaving.

Q. Can we go on to something else? Suppose a child came to you and said they were being ill treated in the home. Would you take what the child said as the truth or would you start your own investigations?

A. Before I acted on anything I would go into it with the residential staff of the home. I wouldn't take the child's word for it. Knowing children they are likely to elaborate and embellish a story, make mountains out of molehills. While we are on the subject most of the children are from broken homes and are not averse to adding a bit to a tale.

Q. What you are saying then is that by virtue of their background they have survived by manipulating situations and will continue to do so until the pattern is broken.

A. Yes.

Q. Often one gets a field worker who says he has been in residential work and got out and wouldn't have the job again at any price. Yet these same people make demands on the residential staff that they themselves couldn't fulfill if they were in the residential worker's position. How do you feel about that?

A. They obviously realised just how hard residential work is for them to get out. If I have a problem I will go and discuss it with the residential staff or talk to the child but after I've done this and I leave I have still left the problem in the home. I may have sorted part of the problem but staff of the home are left to cope with it. I still think I have quite a good relationship with staff in homes and in the main I think they do a good job.

Q. You accept that you have to work hard to establish and maintain good relationships with residential staff.

A. Yes. I think it is nice when staff say to me, "I've a vacancy if you need one". I know then that I must have a good relationship in that home. I am working on a case at present in which there are three children involved. Mother is dead and father is rejecting two of the children. The residential staff think the children would be better if they were fostered and after some discussion over the case I agree with them.. I've told the staff I will try to see the father and if he doesn't want to see me I will go ahead and foster, because at present these children are really missing a Mum and Dad figure.

Q. You don't think that a residential home is a suitable placement for these children?

A. It is not just my opinion, it is a joint decision between myself and the staff of the home. The home is just being used as a holding unit. I'm looking for the right place for these children and the staff of the home understand this. The staff have spoken to me on and off about it and it isn't just a one off thing. We have had some long discussions about it for some months now.

Q. There is another thing comes to mind (and I know it happens) where you get a residential worker who has come into possession of information about a child which could throw a lot of light onto a case and yet they withhold it out of say a misguided sense of confidentiality. Does this upset you?

A. We all hold information back, especially if we think it will be helpful to a child. I hold information back because sometimes I feel if I tell all I know it may prove detrimental to a child. If they think it is going to help the child I don't mind.

Q. But don't you think this would be a form of collusion. I know when I was in residential work and after a case conference had reached a decision a member of staff would come and say, "You should have done so and so" I used to hit the roof when this had happened.

A. Yes, but let's face it, we break the rules all the time. If we were to work strictly according to the book we would get nowhere. Therefore, I think if it is going to benefit a child in the long term fair enough.

Q. When I was in residential work and even now I am of the opinion that when a fieldworker has a difficult client they are often afraid of that client and will resort to all kinds of tricks including bribery to ease the path for themselves and ignore the problems they are creating. How do you feel about this?

A. This sort of thing does happen. If a fieldworker is afraid of someone he should say so and hand the case over to someone else.

Q. Have you any instances of downright bad management on the part of any residential worker in any of your cases.

A. No, but I do think you have to have a balance with staff in the homes. If you have someone who tends to get a bit high then you should have someone who is calm and relaxed. There was one home which didn't have this and it troubled me for a time but the situation has changed now and you can feel it when you visit. There was one home I had a problem with but I think we were all at fault and we sorted it out, in fact quite a good relationship has grown out of it.

Q. Do you as a fieldworker think there are great pressures on residential workers?

A. I'm sure there are. I think they are often badly let down and am of the opinion that there should be more staff on in the evenings when children want to talk as things are now staff don't have the time. You may only have two or even one staff on and they are usually busy bathing or getting supper so if a child wants to talk they can't stop long enough to listen. Although it may not seem much if they are trying to do a good job this places pressure on them and I do feel sorry for them, they must feel very frustrated.

Q. Staffing homes is a nightmare I well know. People just do not want unsocial hours and too many authorities try to get residential care on the cheap. What are your opinions?
A. This is the usual "penny pinching". We take a child into care and we are

supposed to do the best for that child and if it means paying more to get the staff we need then we should be prepared to pay it.

A considerable amount of research into depravation, delinquency etc. has been done in the U.S.A. the results of this have been published in this country, in books and in various social work papers. It is not unusual for these publications to be listed for reading by students on courses and it is quite common to find references to these researches in books written by people in this country. Bawlby in Child Care and the Growth of Love p.182 refers to some work in the U.S.A with family welfare associations and draws three lessons from it, one of which is "Family and Child Welfare is a skilled profession for which workers must be thoroughly trained."

Michael Haltby M.S.W devised a list of skills which residential staff should develop in order to perform their task. This list was first devised by him for use in a residential institution in the U.S.A.

The point I wish to make is this. The U.S.A have an army of social workers which are considered by many to be the highest qualified possibly in the world. Yet if what we read and hear is true juvenile crime has reached epidemic proportions, corruption and organised crime is accepted as a way of life, where parts of society are 'kinky' in the extreme, murder is commonplace and drug trafficking is breaking bounds, where the police are liable to shoot first and ask questions after. Also this is the country which gave us mugging.

Chapter 8

I became involved in residential work in homes for the aged due to changing my job. I took a post in the Training Department of a big authority. It was not long before I discovered that staff in these homes had problems and frustrations very similar to those I had so recently suffered. One major exception was, while one could usually get children to involve themselves in doing small tasks around the home these people were faced with the almost impossible task of getting the aged to do anything, even for their wellbeing. Also, like staff of Children's homes, they were never short of advice about how the job should be done. The following cases and comments are from residential staff of homes for the aged, and I mean staff who live on the premises.

Before I go on, let me draw your attention to something which if you have not visited a part 111 home** you may not be aware of. When you go into a home you will no doubt see a number of elderly of both sexes sitting around in the entrance or the lounges. They look clean, warm and comfortable. Have you ever stopped to think how much care and effort goes into just those three things? The old man or woman you look at may be blind, diabetic, doubly incontinent and unable to walk without assistance from either staff or with the use of a zimmer. He/she may have soiled themselves an hour before you got there and one or two staff will have spent that hour bathing and changing the old person. You may think when you see the residents that they are all nice grandfathers or grandmothers and while I admit that many are nice and will make some effort on their own behalf, there are many who refuse to do anything for themselves and are very cruel, and yes, wicked to other residents and staff.

You may not like or believe what you read in the following pages but I assure you that it happens and after all., that is what this book is about the

** (Part 111 home – A Residential Home for the elderly)

things that people like to pretend do not happen but which is the practical world of the residential social worker.

Before I started to write this section I spoke to a man who was a trained cook and had worked in two homes, one a mixed and the other all female. In the first home he had often helped with the male residents as he was the only male member of staff. He was, incidentally, only two years from retirement himself.

Q. What are your views of working in a part 111 home in terms of someone who is on the periphery of residential work'?

A. I see people come into homes reasonably active and in a short time stagnate. They need some motivation but what kind I don't know as they seem to resist all efforts on the part of the staff. I have found the women worse than the men. I have seen men, even confused ones, make their own beds, maybe not perfectly, but they made the effort. The women seem to be the ones who make the least effort. They come into these homes and they will do nothing despite encouragement from staff. Ask them to do something and they don't want to know. They will tell you it's not their job. They just opt out they will not help a Care Assistant to do even the smallest job. They just sit there and say, "We're keeping you lot". They won't even sit in the garden on a nice summer's day; they will tell you "It's too cold". After a few years they are just cabbages. I have had some who would help me wash up but they soon get tired of it and stop. Surely there must be something more than just sitting in rows watching other people work.

Q. Are you saying there is no encouragement? Is it lack of encouragement or are you saying that when they come into a home they are given the impression that everything will be done for them?

A. I think they are given the impression that everything should be done for them. It is a hard job for any officer in charge to say "they will do this or that" for they will turn around and say "That is what you are here for". Surely if they were in their own place they would keep themselves tidy, make their own beds and, in general make an effort and then they wouldn't be so damned bored. If you organize an outing how many will go? You might get 12 to agree to a day out but when the day comes you have only three and you have to force them to go. They should be encouraged to help themselves.

Q. Surely there is encouragement for residents to participate in all sorts of activities in the home? If they choose not to involve themselves, what do you do?

A.I don't know the answer to that. I was a milkman for 22 years before coming back to cooking and I dealt with old people all that time and they looked after themselves. It was a struggle but they managed. Some were 85 and 90 and they did their bit of shopping some even did a bit of gardening and they managed but they come into homes and they opt out of everything. I don't know what the answer is.[76]

Q. Do you think then that the trend over the last few years has been to do it for them rather than get them to do it for themselves?

A. You could be right. There is something which does disturb me though. There are people who come into care, become ill and can't be kept in these homes and perhaps have to go into hospital. They come here and they are off someone's hands they go to hospital and they are off the Social Services hands. The hospital hand them back as a social problem and they are off their hands. No - one seems to want to know. They are just shuttled about from pillar to post. It's a shame really but I don't know what the answer is.

There was one day and due to sickness, there were only two staff on duty and not one resident offered any help and at least half of them were quite capable and they expected everything to be on time and complained when it wasn't, but help!! - not a chance. The two staff were exhausted at the end of the day. The incontinent ones still had to be toiletted or cleaned up if they had soiled themselves. No-one said to them "You could help". You have only to insist that an old person makes an effort and walk by themselves and have a visitor who knows nothing about the work, see it, and the next thing is you are accused of being cruel to residents. The fact that it may well be for the old person's own good doesn't seem to matter.

There is a section of Society who say that Part 111 homes should be made into extensions of geriatric wards. I have news for them they already are. We have the Purple Book issued by the D.H.S.S. and in it there are several recommendations. Among them are (a)"Medical care should be provided by the Area Health Board with the District Nurse visiting, on the instructions of the Doctor and when requested by the Officer in Charge". (b) "Care should approximate home care of the sick". It does not appear to have occurred to the D.H.S.S. that when a family nurse a sick person at home, it is usually on a 1 to 1 or 1 to 2 basis and often more. We are dealing with a ratio in the region of three residents to one staff and that includes domestics cooks and gardener handymen. If we exclude them, the figure is nearly doubled, always providing all the staff turn in to work which is very rare but more of that later. We are told that ours is a social work function and that we should work towards rehabilitating old people back into Society. A very laudable aim. But, when is a medical problem a social work problem or vice versa? The doctor only has to say "This person is a social problem, I can't get him/her into hospital" and you find it is the residential worker who has to deal with it. Of course having got an old person into Part 111 they will be given medical attention. The D.H.S.S. and others who write pamphlets and booklets etc. on Part 111 residents seem to have missed one rather vital point and that is this _their advice, instructions, whatever you call them are more applicable to the aged who used to be admitted to homes ten to fifteen years ago.

The following is an example of a 40 bedded Home.

There are 12 men and 28 women in residence. One is a diabetic on insulin, three are permanent wheelchair cases one of whom is an amputee, six have to be moved by wheelchair, four are hemiplegics, four blind, three partially sighted, one with multiple sclerosis, one crippled with arthritis, eight have to be dressed, eight mentally confused and one mentally retarded and undergoing psychiatric treatment, two Parkinson's Disease, one with a permanent catheter, six incontinent of urine, one doubly incontinent, seven use zimmer aids and five use other forms of walking aids. The Home also caters for ten day care a week, which means feeding, bathing and washing their clothes. This home was seven staff short due to staff absence, Rehabilitate?? Motivate?? Social Work Function?? I have not mentioned oedema or slightly arthritic or the minor afflictions.

Now, some bright person might add those up and say "This chap is talking rubbish. I've added those up, it comes to 62 and its only a 40 bedded home". If you have done so then you are uninitiated because the residents can, and do, suffer from any one, two, three or more of the illnesses and/or afflictions.[64]

A man, aged 87 fell downstairs backwards and fractured his pelvis. He was taken to hospital and after a few days he was returned to the home with instructions that the staff should immobilize him for two weeks. He was stone deaf, severely confused and doubly incontinent. He kept getting out of bed and falling (staff were of the opinion that he was trying to go to the toilet). He was black and blue all over through falling and staff said he was just like a rag doll. A member of staff who went to check on him found him lying on the floor in faeces and urine. He was again sent to hospital. Two days later, the hospital wanted to return him to the home saying he was much improved. A social problem?[46:49]

Hospital staff can immobilize a patient and no - one will question them. Try doing the same thing in a home and there will be complaints from visitors about cruelty.[44]

An old lady in a home with 22 beds was senile. She could not sit in a chair and kept falling to the floor. Staff were constantly picking her up. To avoid an accident, she had to be strapped into a sitting position at the table. The Officer in Charge spoke to the doctor about her and he said it would be safer if the old lady was left on the floor and propped up with cushions, as she could not fall very far if she was already on the floor. It so happened that one day when there was only the cook and the Officer in Charge on duty, they were trying to get the evening meal ready and set the tables. The Officer in Charge went into the lounge and found this old lady on the floor, so she decided to take the doctor's advice, so that she would be able to help the cook. While she was doing this, a relative of another resident called to visit. The Officer in Charge left the old lady propped up on the floor and went to finish helping to put the meal out. She returned and helped the old lady to her feet and took her into the dining room. Two days later, the Office received an anonymous letter saying how wicked the staff were to residents in this particular home and demanding that the Officer in Charge be dismissed within seven days, or else. The letter was shown to the Officer in Charge, who made it quite plain that she had a good idea who had written the letter and that if the writer, anyone in the office, or the doctor could do any better, she would gladly hand her job over. She also made it known to her seniors that the women the visitor had been to see was noted in the home for her wicked tongue and was constantly causing trouble amongst the other residents and trying to set staff against one another. When the visitor called the next time, the Officer in Charge mentioned the incident of the old lady on the floor to her and also the anonymous letter and that she had her suspicions as to who had written it and that if she could obtain proof, the writers would find themselves facing a court action - the visitor was the soul of discretion and politeness from then on.[45,46,80]

There was an old lady in a 28 bedded home. The home was an adapted property with dormitory type bedrooms. Staff were of the opinion that the lady was dying. She was in bed yet had the strength to get out and usually fell in doing so. She was also hallucinating. The staff were at their wits end as, although they were not trained nurses, they were doing their best to nurse the woman but could not be with her twenty four hours a day. The officer in Charge realized that the situation required more expert advice and telephoned the doctor who asked if it was an emergency. This was *9.15a.m* and at 11 a.m. the doctor had not been, so the Officer in Charge telephoned again, only to be told that he was going to a conference and had to catch a train at 12 noon but would contact the emergency doctor and ask him to call. Time went on and eventually the officer in charge telephoned the emergency doctor herself. He arrived at 3.30p.m and prescribed some form of tranquillizing tablets. The old lady got worse, so the Officer in Charge contacted the doctor again and was told over the phone to increase the dosage. Altogether, the old lady was in bed for ten days before she died. Another social problem? [47][48]

We are told by the D.H.S.S. that nursing duties are not to be performed by the staff of homes, as this will be undertaken by the Area Health Board, but no-one has seen fit to define nursing duties. We can get the situation where the District Nurse will call at a home to put on a dry dressing on an old person. An hour later the old person will have removed it, so staff of the home will have to replace it. Are staff supposed to call the district nurse again, or not'? If they query such a situation they will be told "If it was your mother or father you would do it". I submit if it had been a relative in their own home, the Nurse would not have been called to such a task in the first place. It seems to me that instructions are passed down from the top administrators and legislation goes on the statute book without any thought being given to how they are going to be made to work, or provision being made to this end. It does not appear to have filtered up to the corridors of power that for some years now residential workers have been nursing sick residents under the guidance of the doctor and if the doctor felt the situation warranted it, the District Nurse would be instructed to attend and assist, or advise. Are we now going to move towards a situation where the special relationship between the doctor and residential staff working to the same end is to be destroyed? Are we now to get our homes losing the personal touch due to bureaucracy? [47:81]

There was a home with four residents in bed ill. Three of them had fractured shoulders. The District Nurse attended once a week to attend to one of those with a fractured shoulder. The staff had to attend to the resident for the rest of the time and also the other three who were in bed. The Officer in Charge asked the Nurse about the others. She said she had no idea there were any others in the same position and had no instructions regarding them. They had also been to hospital. Residential staff can be forgiven for wondering if hospital staff and doctors in particular have been acquainted with the latest instruction. There is no appeal against a doctor's decision,[48] except to another doctor, which only generates ill feeling. Such situations culminate in the Officer in Charge of a home having to take a stand and risk accusations of being uncaring when, in point of fact, it is more often the opposite.

An old woman of 90 was found unconscious on a lounge floor. Upon questioning the other residents, the Officer in Charge could only conclude she had suffered some kind of fit. When she was picked up, she appeared to have a left side hemiplegia. The Officer in Charge telephoned the doctor who sent an ambulance. There was no time to write down details for the driver and he was acquainted with the details verbally. Two hours later, the staff nurse telephoned the Officer in Charge and said they were returning the old lady as the doctor was happy with her condition. The Officer in Charge queried this and refused to have the old lady until she had at least been kept for overnight observation. The result was the old lady was found to be very ill, the hospital said she kept having fits which they could not explain. A few days later the Deputy telephoned the hospital to enquire about their resident and was told she was no better. A short time later the old lady died and no - one saw fit to inform the home, though her bed was being held against her return. The Residents Committee of the home were very distressed when they were told as it was their practice to send flowers to the funeral of anyone from the home.

There was an old lady in a 40 bedded home. Staff had spoken to the doctor about her and he was of the opinion that she should be seen by a Psychiatrist. He said he would arrange it. Two days later the doctor told the officer that he had spoken to the psychiatrist and they would expect him anytime. The woman was in the habit of defecating wherever she was, in the lounge, in the dining room, bed etc. She would also smear faeces all over herself. She was also in the habit of hiding food about her person, in her bra, up her clothes and distributing it to the other residents. Staff were worried stiff because her hands were contaminated with faeces and they were finding it increasingly difficult to keep her clean, as she could not be watched every minute of the day and toileting at regular intervals was proving to be fruitless. This went on for some weeks until eventually, about half the residents took ill and were confined to bed. I leave you to imagine the problems for staff having to nurse about twenty sick old people and I am not counting the others who had to be cared for.[64] The doctor was called in. He alerted the Area Health Board and the Environmental Health Dept, who suspected food poisoning. Tests were made and within twenty four hours, the old lady was moved to a Psychiatric Unit. The sick residents recovered albeit slowly but one shudders at the possible outcome and I am prepared to bet there were a number of people who heaved very deep sighs of relief.

Many residential staff working with the aged say they keep residents who should be in hospital because if they send one into hospital they more often than not get one in a worse condition in return. I know a man who is an Officer in Charge of a home and during his earlier career he worked in a hospital on a male geriatric ward. He admitted to me quite frankly that it was quite common practice to arrange for the more 'troublesome' patients be sent to a Part 111 home on the premise that if they kept the 'best' life was that much easier for the hospital. This in spite of the fact that residential workers are not supposed to perform nursing duties, or that they do not have the same facilities as a hospital and also, in many cases, staff of homes do not have nursing or medical qualifications to cater for such residents. An Officer in Charge went to a hospital to assess a prospective resident (a woman). The Officer in Charge was chatting to the woman for a few moments when a chance remark triggered off severe aggression and the woman became very violent towards the Officer in Charge who had been on the point of accepting her. The Officer in Charge came to the conclusion that the woman was mentally unbalanced. The Charge Nurse said the woman was ready to go out. The Hospital Social Worker witnessed the incident and supported the Officer in Charge in refusing to take the woman. From this, it was discovered that the woman was on Largactil as required, though this was not on the medical record which had been given to the Officer in Charge.

A district nurse went to a home to attend to a resident who she had been told had been admitted from hospital. The nurse asked for the new resident by name. The Officer in Charge told her that they had no one of that name in the home and asked if she was sure she had the right name and had come to the right home. The Nurse left and a few hours later an ambulance drew up at the door with the new resident. The Officer in Charge knew nothing about a new admission. The nurse was contacted and came right away. This was early evening. The new resident had no medical records and only a sealed letter to the G.P. The Officer in Charge and the nurse opened the letter and found that the resident was a diabetic and the letter gave the insulin dosage and nothing else. The nurse telephoned to get more information and was told the next injection was due the following morning. It was also noticed in the letter that the dosage had been altered and the original dose was lower than that which was required. The Officer in Charge contacted the dietician at the hospital and asked for a diet sheet for the resident for obvious reasons. The resident had to go back into hospital after two weeks and the Officer in Charge never did get the diet sheet. The same Officer in Charge commented on the time the new resident arrived at the home and he said "Residents who are brought to the home during early evening or late afternoon get no time to settle in". When complaints are made to the hospital about this, staff are told the ambulance crews are to blame and so the wheel goes on turning.[50]

One Officer in Charge called the doctor and an ambulance to a man of 66 who had suffered a coronary. The man was in an upstairs room. The doctor arrived before the ambulance and on seeing the man said he needed oxygen and asked why there wasn't any in the home, stressing the fact that homes should have some. When the ambulance arrived, the crew said they did not have mobile oxygen on the vehicle. It was decided to carry the sick man downstairs. The Officer in Charge commented forcibly on how ridiculous the situation was and the futility of calling the ambulance. One of the ambulance men said he would carry the oxygen cylinder up to the sick man but by the time they got it to him it was too late, the man had died.

There was a man of 78 who was unable to pass water. The Officer in Charge contacted the doctor, who said the man needed be catheterized and asked the Officer in Charge to arrange it with the District Nursing Service. The Officer was told they were unable to help as there was no male nurse available. The

Officer was told they would take the man in to insert the catheter provided they were given a firm promise that the home would take him back. The Officer in Charge said he was of the opinion that the resident was too ill to be moved. The Nursing Service agreed to send someone. Two female nurses arrived and one said she would try and insert the catheter and succeeded. The nurse returned next morning and was told that the resident had passed no water but was passing blood. The Officer told the nurse she was wasting time and that the resident should be in hospital but the nurse said she would have to seek guidance. While she was away, the man died. The doctor was called and certified death. As the doctor left, the nurse returned saying they were to remove the catheter, only to be told it was too late.

The same Officer in Charge was told by a locum doctor (when his own doctor was away) that he could not get a resident into hospital as it would spoil his chances of getting one of his own patients in.

There was a woman of 84. She had a fall and was taken to hospital. A week later the hospital contacted the home and said they were returning her. She arrived in an ambulance and was brought into the home on a stretcher. She had been catheterized. Staff put her to bed immediately and were of the opinion that she was dying, which she did a day or two later. The Coroner's Officer called on the Officer in Charge regarding the death of the old lady and intimated that the hospital had said she was quite alright when she left them. The Officer in Charge was most upset at this and recounted the circumstances of the woman's readmission also their opinions at the time. The Coroner's Officer was told that the body was still on the premises if he wished to see it and make his own assessment. When he saw the body he said "My God" and something which sounded like "I'll have something to say about this". The Officer of the home never heard another word about the case.

There are good and bad in every walk of life and genuine residential staff get very distressed when faced with the situations I have related in this chapter.

Taken For A Ride- Michael Meacher

(45) Mrs. Howlett spent every day strapped into a geriatric chair and was very often to be seen with her head on her crooked elbow slumped over the tray which was locked into the chair. She only rarely uttered any words and when she did so, they were expressed in a slow and very indistinct drawl. Yet when an effort was made to communicate with her, she showed she could think logically and construct short rational sentences. Her husband had died of cancer three years previously, as a result of which she became very depressed (as the case record makes clear), lived an isolated life and refused to mix. Her son and his wife, however, built two rooms on to her bungalow at their own expense and came to look after her. But because she still proved very trying and had lost interest in herself, the daughter—in—law soon collapsed under the strain and was forced to return to her parents home to recuperate. Since the son was also subject to bouts of depression, Mrs. Howlett was admitted informally to the nearby mental hospital where she appeared restless and confused, continually wandering around in an aimless manner and demanding constant attention from the nursing staff.

(48) Little evidence would be assembled on this important subject, but the implications of the limited data were disquieting. In only one of the separist homes were residents encouraged to choose(or retain) their own doctor, but more important were the problems confused residents encountered in communicating the genuineness and urgency of their complaints to staff as requiring a doctor's visit:

A woman of eighty-eight who was disoriented, tangenital in speech and subject to excessive fiddling (score 8) complained at the time of my visit of sharp pains in her back. The staff were openly suspicious of the reality of this alleged imposition and assured her somewhat flippantly that she would soon be better. At her interview she protested bitterly at this indifference: "I wish the doctor would come - pain in my back and all over. I want to go somewhere where somebody knows more about my back. My back is a misery. I'd like a change now. I'd like to go to Furleigh Hospital and see what they can do". Despite her pleas and periodical groaning, the matron did not finally call the doctor till several days had elapsed.

(64) Data already presented has demonstrated the staffing shortage, on a weighted basis, in the separist homes (Table 8.5) and at least in one such home exceptionally long, but fewer, shifts of twelve hours were opted for by married women staff, despite the likely decline in care standards caused by tiredness, because they offered longer unbroken periods of time - off. But apart from the pressure of work and the effects of exhaustion, it may also be surmised that the comparative lack of rational observers in the special homes might undermine staff inhibitions against rougher or less sensitive handling of the confused at times of frustration because of their vague or slow reactions.

Residential Work with the Elderly. C. Paul Brearley

(44) Hospitals are concerned primarily with treatment of illness and disease and with returning the individual to a state of good health and to his normal community roles and with limiting the disabling effects of impairment. Long - term hospital care will have to be provided for some elderly patients who are very infirm or suffering from chronic illness and a need a degree of nursing care that is unavailable elsewhere. Normally this means that social support networks in the community are inadequate or non - existent; most families do provide good, concerned care for elderly relatives, sometimes to the point of exhaustion and collapse. Those hospitals and wards that provide long term care share similar goals to those of residential accommodation, of meeting individual needs for a degree of stimulation, satisfaction and contentment.

(46) Both passive and active overt violence clearly result when staff have little support, poor training and are under pressures of overwork and overcrowding as well as working in a low - status position.

(47) Miller and Gwynne (1972) have proposed two models of residential care which define the primary task of a residential institution in rather different ways. They suggest a warehousing model, in which the primary task is seen as the prolongation of human life, and a horticultural model, in which the primary task is seen as the development of the unsatisfied needs, drives, and unfulfilled capacities of the deprived individuals who live in care.

Although in many ways a helpful categorization this does not take into account the fact that each member of staff and each resident or patient will have an individual view of the goals and tasks of the home or hospital. The way in which the formal organization of the institution is constituted will relate to the overt objectives, the stated aims of the hospital, home etc. The ways in which it actually functions and operates on a day - to - day basis will be more closely linked to the unspoken objectives of individuals which may well vary from one moment to the next.

(49) A ministry memorandum (Ministry of Health 1965) to local authorities and hospitals set out broad categories of older people for whom they might normally expect to have to provide accommodation. It also suggested that the right way to deal with those who were wrongly placed was to accept the status quo for those already in care but to try to avoid wrong placement in the future by joint planning.

(50) The social worker's role lies in smoothing the practicalities of admission and in helping the client towards a realistic handling of fantasies.

Preparing the home - the residential worker's role.

The last mentioned difficulty of the field worker in handing over a client exists as a difficulty also for the residential worker. It is often hard to share clients but it is important for the smoother arrangement of admission that field and residential can collaborate. Just as it is important for the client to visit the home it may in some situations be important for the residential worker to visit the old person in his/her home before admission. Whether this is useful for a particular client must be a matter for discussion between field worker, client and residential worker:

Some clients feel happier if they can meet the new worker on safe ground where they feel able to present their whole personality. The field worker's assessment must be available to the residential worker who must know how to follow up existing a treatment programme, or how to modify it and, in the short term, how to prepare the home for the client. Preparations will be on the practical level and on individual and group levels in the home. The new resident should feel he/she is expected and welcomed; the fears and fantasies about the home will only be exaggerated by inadequate preparation for arrival:

Residential Care Reviewed P.S.S.C. 1977

(76) It is a sound principal however to work towards enabling a resident to leave the home. It encourages residents to use their capabilities to the full in response to what is expected of them. For those who wish to leave, particularly young handicapped people, the possibility of returning; or moving out for the first time to the community should not only be maintained and encouraged, but practical opportunities should also be created. Preparation for this eventuality is as important as that for admission, because considerable help may be needed to enable a resident to live independently. Those homes which provide trial units or flats on their own premises allow the residents to try living independently before moving out. In this way he/she can gain experience in shopping, cooking and cleaning for themselves.

(80) Complaints procedures will differ according to the providing body but we draw attention to the report of the Davies committee on hospital complaints procedure (1973) in which the following basic criteria are laid down:

1. Arrangements should allow the free flow of suggestions or complaints by patients, their relatives or friends.

2. Procedures for dealing with suggestions and complaints should be well – known and easily accessible to all; comprehensive and credible, and fair and just to all concerned.

3. Initial investigation and satisfaction of complaints should be by management, but there should be provision for independent, external review of all complaints.

(81) The selection of the right person for senior posts is obviously crucial and too a great extent must depend primarily on his/her understanding of the work and his/her personal qualities. The professional qualifications he/she will need, while depending on the policies adopted by his/her employing authority for the provision of skills, are those which will have trained him/her to understand his/her duty and to be able to pass on that understanding to his/her team. A nursing qualification is not essential since nursing skills can be called in, although it may be appropriate; but a residential social worker qualification is highly desirable. Training courses linked to the policy needs of the local authority can be very helpful, and in this respect in service training schemes are valuable for relating training to immediate needs.

Procedures for considering applications and allocating places should be established on the basis of joint decision making by people with different skills and knowledge.

Chapter 9

T here seems to be an abysmal ignorance of the role of Part 111 homes. People, who should know better, will ring a home and ask for the Warden. Residential homes mean just that. They are home to the aged in care, yet some authorities still allow the iniquitous "Swap" system, which means that an old person may not have any security of tenure in the only home they have.[51] If we take the last case, would any hospital return a dying person to their home if that home was in an ordinary street with only relatives to cater for the dying person's needs. If a person in their own home was in need of hospital treatment, would the doctor insist on putting someone in the prospective patient's home before agreeing to admit? It would also seem that many hospital social workers need to have the role of Part 111 homes made clear to them and what the various types of homes have to offer. [83]

There was a woman of 70 in an adapted home with no lift. She needed a short stay in hospital for treatment and it was said only two weeks. The Hospital Social Worker telephoned the Officer in Charge and said the Consultant Geriatrician wanted to put a patient in the home in place of the resident he was taking. The Officer in Charge told the Social Worker that the room was the resident's and that it was not right that a complete stranger should be allowed amongst her personal belongings for two weeks —even staff would not be allowed to touch anything while a resident was away. Also, it was against policy to "swap". Half an hour later, the Hospital Social Worker telephoned again and said the woman would not be coming back and again asked for the bed. The Officer in Charge said the policy had not changed in so short a time. She checked with her immediate superiors who supported her decision. The next day, the doctor telephoned a very senior officer. No-on knows what was said but word came down to admit the patient from hospital. The Officer went against his own laid down policy. Six weeks later, the resident who was not supposed to be coming out of hospital was discharged to another home amongst strangers, as all the beds in her original home had been filled.

The Officer in Charge of the home went to the hospital to assess the prospective resident and asked the Ward Sister if the old lady could climb stairs as all the beds she had were in an upstairs bedroom. The Sister replied, "Oh you people are all the same, if their face doesn't fit you don't want them, we can't choose our patients". The Officer in Charge was annoyed at this attitude and told the Sister that personal appearances had nothing to do with it but she knew what physical shortcomings the home had and if an old person could not cope with them, they would be in a continual state of stress and that was the only criteria for accepting or refusing a new resident. The Sister took the Officer to see the old lady and the Officer in Charge repeated her query about climbing stairs. The Sister said she could and they would take her down to Physiotherapy so the Officer in Charge could see for herself. There were three steps up and three steps down with a handrail on both sides. The old lady negotiated these with some difficulty. The Officer in Charge was not too happy about the old lady's ability but said to the Sister "Alright, I'll take your word and admit her". As she was leaving, the Sister said to her, "I wouldn't trust your seniors if I were you my dear". The new resident arrived and was assisted into the home. She took one look at the staircase with balustrades six feet apart and said to the Officer in Charge, "Do I have to go up there!! "I'm afraid so", said the Officer in Charge. The old lady sat down and started weeping, at the same time voicing her inability to do so. At this time, the old lady's son arrived to see her, having heard that she was to be admitted. When he was acquainted with situation, he became very angry and declared his intention of taking the matter up. He either had some influence or frightened some officials, as his mother was moved to another home the next day. As it was, an old lady was subjected to a traumatic experience and a very unhappy twenty four hours. [85]

It would save a lot of ill feeling if hospital staff on Geriatric Wards and Hospital Social Workers were required to visit Part 111 homes to see what facilities they have to offer. I admit that student nurses do, in the course of their training, visit homes but by the time they have reached a position of authority; the situation they saw will have changed or will have become very dim in their minds. Both sides for instance seem to have different ideas of mobility in a patient/resident. A patient in hospital my be able to walk from their bed with or without aid, to the toilet at the end of the ward. In a home, although the toilets and dining room may be close to the lounges, the bedroom they occupy may well be at the other side of the building and the old person may be unable to negotiate the distance without maximum aid from staff. Hospital staff either fail, or refuse to realise that a residential home is totally different to a hospital situation.

There was a man of 78 in a 30 bedded home. All single rooms. The General Practitioner had diagnosed pneumonia, he fell out bed continually, staff checked regularly to see he was alright. The District Nurse called to see him and suggested someone sat with him all the time. The staff had to explain to her that there were another 29 people to be cared for. In a ward situation, a nurse can see all her patients but the same does not apply in a home. The consultant came to see this particular man with the view of admitting him to hospital. At the time, the man was on a ripple bed. The consultant said he had nothing to offer and refused to admit the man. "Anyway", said the consultant, "this is a welfare home and an institution". I cannot think of anything which would annoy residential staff more than a comment such as that. However, the resident died a few days later and after he had died, the hospital telephoned the home and offered to take him on an exchange basis.

Residential staff rightly complain that they are misled by hospitals over information and the ability of a prospective resident and, on occasions, receive no information at all and, [84] having admitted the patient, found they could not cope, will meet with a flat refusal if they want to return the old person to hospital. I have spoken to many Officers in Charge before starting this book and not one could remember when the hospital told them that a prospective resident was incontinent and often the old person is doubly so. Officers say if they ask the hospital whether the prospective resident is incontinent, they will be told "No' yet when they take such as this up with the hospital, they will be told "They were alright when they left us".[52:53] What is even more surprising, I have heard of social workers telling people in the community that an elderly relative could not be admitted to a Part 111 home because they did not take incontinents.

An old man was admitted to a residential home. After a while he became incontinent and was continually falling and hurting himself. The G.P. finally got him into the hospital and the Officer in Charge called the next day to assess another prospective resident. Whilst he was in hospital, he asked how the old man was and was told by the Geriatrician that it would be 10 to 12 weeks before the man would be able to return. Two days later, the Hospital Social Workers contacted the Officer in Charge and said they were returning the old man as he was alright. The Officer in Charge asked if they had suddenly developed a miracle cure as two days earlier the man had been seriously ill. The Social Worker said she would ring back. Ten minutes later she rang back to say the Geriatrician said the man had just had a relapse.[85]

There was an old lady with a broken humerous. She had been attended to in hospital and they announced their intention of sending her home. The Social Worker would not agree to this as she was of the opinion that the old lady would not be able to manage. The doctor insisted that the old lady would have to be discharged. The Social Worker arranged for the old lady to be admitted to Part 111 for a short time and within ten minutes of going to the home, the old lady dropped dead.

Far too often, old people who are to be admitted to residential care are given no information about their intended placement, or they are told they are going to a place where everything will be done for them.

A Geriatrician contacted a Senior Social Worker with a view to putting a 58 year old hemiplegic man into a home. Although the man was by no means old, it was agreed he would be admitted. In view of the situation, it was agreed that a Field Worker would accompany the Officer in Charge to the hospital to see the man. They were met at the door by the Geriatrician and the Hospital Social Worker. The Officer in Charge met the man and was very surprised to find the man knew nothing about his intended move. The Officer in Charge spoke to the

Ward Sister about it and she told him that no - one had, at any time, discussed the move with man, who refused point blank to go to any other home than his own. An attempt was made by the Officer in Charge to persuade the man to change his mind but without success. The Geriatrician and the Hospital Social Worker were acquainted with the situation and said "Well, we will just have to keep him". The Officer in Charge and the Field Worker had driven a twenty mile round trip, which had been a complete waste of time. One wonders if the Geriatrician and the Hospital Social Worker saw the man as a human being or, perhaps, they made the same mistake many make, namely, assuming that a person who is handicapped must also be mentally deficient.[85:86]

The following case may well be regarded as something of a digression but I think it serves to illustrate the attitude of some so called caring professionals towards old people.

There was an old lady of 90 in a Private Home for the Aged She took ill and the Proprietor called the doctor, who said he could not get the resident into hospital, as there was no room and old people were having to sleep on mattresses on the floor. The Proprietor's wife had been a nursing auxiliary and told the doctor not to take them for complete fools and indicated she thought he had no intention of trying to get the old lady into the hospital. She also pointed out to the doctor that neither she nor her husband, were qualified nurses. For seven days and nights the couple took it in turns to look after the resident, who was confined to bed. Finally, the hospital consented to take her. She was dressed and sent to hospital late one morning. She was returned at 1.10a,m. the next morning. It was freezing and snowing and the Proprietor was shocked to find the only thing the woman had on were her knickers. She was brought in with a blanket wrapped around her. The ambulance man took the old lady into the lounge, refused to assist in getting her to her bedroom, even though she could only walk with the aid of a zimmer.

There is a section of the community who regard old people as just dead meat, something which has outlived its usefulness and not really worth bothering about. The following case drove the Officer in Charge to leave the authority.

There was a lady of 80+. She was a single amputee, also diabetic and although slightly confused, she was very lively and had a good appetite. The Officer in Charge noticed the old lady was going off her food and it was suspected that diabetes was the cause. The G.P. was called and the staff of the home were of the opinion that this particular man was carrying on a private vendetta against Social Services, as he never examined a patient and just referred them to hospital. This he did to the old lady referring her to the Diabetic Clinic. The tests proved negative and the old lady was taken again a month later for a further checks which again proved negative. The old lady gradually got worse. It was fortunate she had her own bedroom though she still kept the whole corridor awake. Staff were having to take it in turns at sitting with her night and day and they say she had a frightened, haunted look in her eyes, as if she was going crazy (staffs' description, not mine). Staff found the only way to comfort the woman was to hold her hand and sing to her. The G.P. was called again and did nothing. He was finally pressed to call in a Geriatrician, who said it was not his field and that the lady should be seen by a Psychiatrist. The Psychiatrist called a week later and said it was the Geriatrician's field. Each one tried to pass the ball to the other. All this time, the old lady became more confused and her condition continued to deteriorate. Eventually, she contracted a chest infection and staff could not persuade her to take any food. The G.P.was called again on Tuesday and did not attend until Thursday. When he saw the old lady he called the emergency ambulance to take her to hospital, where she died two days later. The Officer in Charge felt that the old lady was 'snatched' from them at the last minute, as, had she been left to die in the home, two days would not have made a great deal of difference, as it had been going on for <u>four months!!</u> All the hospital were concerned about was how soon they could put someone else in her place. The Officer in Charge had offered to take "a swap" a few weeks beforehand, in order to get treatment for her resident but the doctor had resisted any attempt to admit from Part 111. The Officer in Charge felt no- one but the staff of the home cared at all. I have said that residential staff complain that they often prefer to keep a sick resident, even though hospital treatment may be needed because, if they agree to "swap" the new resident is often worse than the old.[85] I often wonder if this is not the old workhouse philosophy where conditions inside were deliberately made so appalling that people would sooner suffer terrible hardship in the community than go into such an institution which benefited the administering body as it reduced the numbers they had to provide for.

There was an old man of 80, he was doubly incontinent and could only walk with staff help. He was completely unable to stand alone. As he kept falling across the table at mealtimes, staff had to provide him with a table or his own, as it was also upsetting other residents to see his condition. He was also a smoker and staff had to be constantly alert as he could not hold his cigarette. I understand the medical term for his condition is "catalepsy". The doctor recommended hospital and arranged for his admission. It was agreed it could be a "swap". The hospital wanted the Officer in Charge to take a man who was a permanent wheelchair case, who could not get out of bed on his own and needed attention during the night because of this. He also needed toileting during the day. The Officer in Charge decided they might just as well keep their own resident, even though he was obviously a geriatric case. As one member of staff commented, "In spite of what the D.H.S.S. say, this man requires twenty four hours solid nursing". Not only that but the hospital refusal to take the man without a swap meant a bed, which would be of some use to some poor old person in the community was effectively blocked.

By judicious manipulation, the hospital can end up with two beds instead of one. The following shows how this is done.

An old lady was admitted to hospital and died within two days. A week later the hospital contacted the home and said they were sending one of their patients in place of the resident they had taken. That left them with a vacant bed. Simple but clever.

Taken for a Ride- Michael Meacher

(52) Either the relatives 'play it cool' regarding their parents' real mental condition, or else the admissions officer cannot afford the necessary time or make another visit. But it has been one's frequent experience to admit a resident who has been described as 'mildly confused' and to find that it has been necessary to arrange for him to be seen by a consultant psychiatrist who has no hesitation in recommending the patient's immediate removal to the mental hospital. Also it is not unknown for a general practitioner to co-operate in describing a patient as 'mildly confused' in order to get a particularly awkward person off his hands.

Residential work with the elderly – C. Paul Brearley

(51) Artificial, essentially administrative, barriers may also exist, hindering progress through the caring system. Sometimes sick people in residential care can only be moved to hospital in exchange for a patient waiting for transfer; this form of body swapping leads to hurried transfers, often leaving the elderly people concerned confused, disorientated, dissatisfied and far from home. Local problems of distrust between workers in the field, in hospital, and in the home may also build up as a result of a few mistakes or mishandled exchanges. Elitist thinking on the part of groups of workers is also inclined to lead to splitting up of functions; elitist approaches, inevitably leave the elderly consumer at the bottom of the pile. Until administrative barriers can me made more flexible in policy term, and in terms of worker relationships, the continuum of caring approaches cannot be used appropriately to meet individual needs in the correct way. Each elderly person should be at the right place in the system for his own needs, at the right time. One way to encourage this is for workers to be able to function as a team to put consumer need before their own divisive needs.

(53) Geriatric medicine is concerned perhaps as much with the continuing management of illness and future health care of elderly patients as with

the treatment of presenting illness. This concern inevitably extends to the social and emotional needs of the individual patient who can only remain independent in terms of his total internal and external environment.

Preparing the client – the geriatric team.

One important way of overcoming some of the difficulties that have been described is by making adequate, careful preparation before admission. This will involve the worker in the community in making a full assessment of client needs in order to be sure that admission is the best course of action and in discussion and clarification of the implications of admission to build up strengths before the event. If the problems of the elderly are multi – symptomatic then the "solutions" to those problems will best be found by a team of workers both in the community and in the hospital or residential environment. Social workers, health visitors, nurses, general practitioners and hospital doctors all become involved with the older person and his family and friends. Considerable change is often brought about in client's lives by team intervention and it is important to be aware of the implications of the intervention of the geriatric team for social change.

Residential Care Reviewed P.S.S.C. 1977

(83) We emphasize what is said here. Great stress is caused by the fact that admissions to hospital are frequently refused except on an exchange basis. This is because some hospitals assume that homes are equipped to care adequately for the very frail and that this is their proper task. But few homes have planned provision for them, and the practice serves only to highlight the gap in provision. This is a matter on which the general practitioner's judgment is crucial, and it can often require strong action on his part to prevent a person being inappropriately placed by a transfer.

(84) Where background information is to be shared with relevant agencies, this should be made clear to the individual concerned, and reasons

should be given. The purpose for which information (e.g. medical details) is required should be explained and adhered to, and it is important that only strictly relevant details are recorded. There may be occasions when it is in the best interests of the client for certain issues to be discussed without his knowledge, but we advocate his full participation wherever possible and that his consent should be obtained where this can be done.

(85) Throughout this process, the needs and wishes of the client should be of primary importance, however great the pressures to give priority to other considerations. Inevitably there may have to be some compromise, but this should be with the needs and wishes of other clients and not merely for the sake of administrative convenience. The client and/or his family should be kept informed of all procedures and the reasons for all actions taken, and be consulted fully at every stage. Hard-pressed social workers may find this difficult and demanding and there is a danger of accepting decisions which are arbitrary. But careful consultation should take place both for the immediate well being of the client, and to form the basis of his future attitude to residential care.

(86) 'Too often the old person is rushed into care with no thought as to how they feel about it, their home is broken up and their bits and pieces which could have been brought with them scattered'. (Staff) Careful preparation for admission is essential. The client must have time to adapt to the idea of entering a home, to gain a realistic picture of what it entails, and to discuss his anxieties.

Chapter 10

What do staff of homes do in cases like the following?

An old lady in a home was very ill. The doctor called and agreed that she was in need of hospital treatment (to avoid future confusion I will call her Mrs. White). The hospital agreed to take her as a swap. They said they had a patient (we will call Mrs. Brown) who needed a period of rehabilitation before she was returned to her home. Mrs. White went into hospital and Mrs. Brown was admitted to the home. After ten days the hospital contacted the Officer in Charge and told him that Mrs. White would not be returning and asked him to let them know when he thought Mrs. Brown could go home. The staff of the home worked hard with Mrs. Brown and after two months the officer in charge contacted the hospital and told them he was of the opinion she was ready to go home. He said to them, "Give us another month and we will have her setting bricks". The Consultant took Mrs. Brown back into hospital and announced their intention of returning Mrs. White. The Officer in Charge was very surprised and queried her condition. Being denied a satisfactory answer he insisted on seeing her before agreeing to re admit. When he saw Mrs. White in hospital he told the Consultant that he was of the opinion that she was worse than when she was first sent to them and he refused to take her back until there was considerable improvement. The next thing the Officer in Charge heard was that he would be getting a resident from another home (we will call her Mrs. Black). After she had been in the home a few days, the Officer in Charge had a talk with her. He was very annoyed when he was told that she had not wanted to come and had been very happy in the first home. The Officer rang the Officer responsible for moving Mrs. Black and asked what was going on, repeating what Mrs. Black had said. The reply he got was not satisfactory to him and he said he intended to take the matter further. Within two days, Mrs.

Black was taken back to her original home. He was told by the hospital that he would have to take Mrs. White back as she was his resident and there was a gentle hint that beds might be short in future. He found out some weeks later that Mrs. Brown had not been sent home, she was still in the hospital!!!

I must confess I find it appalling that "professionals" barter human beings and excuse it by saying "well, they are at the end of their lives and they've had a good innings". One hears howls of rage when politicians use people as pawns in political power games and in truth some politicians will "raise Cain" when incidents become public knowledge. Yet, the same people who display righteous indignation remain strangely mute at what is happening under their very noses. There is an omnipotent indifference which makes the prospect for us, the elderly of tomorrow, frightening.[56]

One Officer in Charge remarked to me "Hospitals seem to develop a mental block when you ask for a bed and mention the age of a resident. Basically, they just don't want geriatrics".

Hospital staff will tell homes staff that a prospective resident is only mildly confused yet, when the old person is admitted to the home, staff find that they are so confused they will be running around the home naked. Often residents become very distressed at the mental and physical state of admissions from hospital and I think a lot of this distress is caused by fear, fear of what is going to happen to them. The current D.H.S.S. guidelines are instrumental in causing a conflict of objectives. One home I visited had a G.P who said to the Officer in Charge "You can't cope with cases like this in these circumstances, I will contact the hospital". The Consultant went to the home, looked around and said, "You will have to cope with these nursing cases". There were no trained nurses on the staff and he was admitting that those he had seen were nursing cases.

Staff I have spoken to have nothing but praise for the District Nurses yet, here again we also have a conflict of objectives. A nurses's job is purely medical, to nurse the sick and help them back to health. The Residential Workers's job, we are constantly reminded is Social Work, a function which is geared to keeping people mentally and, where possible, physically alert and active. Let me quote an example.

A District Nurse visited a home to attend to a resident. The home was an old adapted property with no lift. The nurse, having attended to the patient, was going through the hall on her way out when she met an old lady struggling along with a zimmer. The Nurse said "My dear, you shouldn't have to struggle like that, you should have a wheelchair". After she had left, the old lady demanded the staff get her a wheelchair and told them they were being very cruel to her, at the same time repeating what the Nurse had said. The home did not lend itself to the use of wheelchairs, even though staff admitted it would be easier for them but, as many who read this will have been told, this is not the object.

I mentioned at the beginning of this section three states, warmth, cleanliness and comfort. It is surprising how little people bother to learn about homes, even those who go into homes on a voluntary basis regularly. Some will even take small children to them and allow the children to run around unsupervised, often a potential danger to old people whom they might run into.

A young woman who had been going into a home twice a week for about eight months as a voluntary worker. She went in during the afternoon, served tea to the residents and chatted to them. A vacancy arose in the home for a part time Care Assistant. The woman approached the Officer in Charge and asked if she could have the job but said that she was not able to do any heavy lifting. The Officer in Charge told her she would not be able to do the work and tried to explain what the job entailed The woman said, "Of course. I would be able to do it. After all I have served tea and biscuits to them"!! She had been going into the home all that time and was blind to the physical and mental state of the residents and fondly imagined that all staff had to do was to serve tea and biscuits.

I know of one home where a voluntary group had to be banned. This was due to some of them providing sweets for diabetic residents. This, in spite of repeated requests by the Officer in Charge not to do so. It only came to light by chance and after great problems had been encountered trying to stabilize the diabetics and the doctor and Officer in Charge worrying why all the treatments were having no effect. The group refused to believe that they were slowly killing these residents.

A young woman was employed in a home as a Care Assistant. It was apparent within a few weeks that she was not going to be suitable and it was thought from what she said that she must have been on some sort of course. She usually managed to bath residents who were capable of bathing themselves and would boast to other staff about how many she had done. The Officer in Charge told her that the object of the exercise was to help those who could not help themselves and instructed her to bath certain residents who required maximum help e.g. lifting in and out. Nothing daunted this woman after this experience was always "busy talking to the residents" when bathing was to be done. She was told about her attitude to the job and replied "I thought we were supposed to stimulate and motivate residents". The Officer in Charge asked her how she thought the rest of the work got done (this home had ten incontinent residents out of a total of 28). The Officer in Charge agreed that stimulation and motivation were part of the job but residents had to be kept clean, warm and comfortable and that toileting, cleaning up faeces, changing clothes and keeping the home clean were also very much part of the caring function and if she would make a proper effort to help the rest of the staff, they could all go and spend some time with the residents. Matters came to a head when the Officer in Charge heard her cursing an old lady with a zimmer, who was struggling to the dining room. She was also seen to push the old lady on several occasions. She was dismissed and the next thing to be heard about it was a letter from the Union. The woman had been to see the representative and alleged cruelty and stated that residents were left alone all day.

New staff, course tutors, a section of the public and also many Social Services employees who should know better, talk very glibly about motivating residents and keeping them active. These people would be more use to residential work if they took the trouble to learn just how frail are the old people who are currently being cared for in Part 111 homes. From the information I have gathered, the majority of old people in homes do not want to be motivated, in fact, some just want to go to bed and stay there.

When a home has half a dozen residents who are incontinent and will defecate where they stand, someone has to clean up and someone has to bath and change the resident. When experienced staff insist that a resident makes an effort, however small, they are open to all sorts of criticism. It can be done in hospital because there, it is a totally different regime. Old people grew up in an era when absolute trust was placed in the doctor and the nurse and whatever these people say is accepted without question. They hold what I call "positional influence". On the other hand, Part 111 homes grew out of those appalling institutions _ the workhouses and they are still viewed with a great deal of suspicion by prospective residents, who probably think that because the treadmill cannot be seen does not mean it is not there and any attempt to involve them in a physical activity is seen as the "thin end of the wedge"

While in the process of gathering material for this work, I went into a home run by a very forward looking Officer in Charge, who was incidentally a S.R.N. up to 18 months before I started to write. This Officer took great pride in the mobility of her residents, the low incidence of confusion and incontinence, also the number of activities in the home. When I went in she said to me "I'm sorry Mr. Taylor would you come some other time please? I have a resident who for four weeks now has been defecating everywhere, on other people's beds, bedroom floors, sinks and waste paper bins and she has just soiled the bedroom of a mentally alert resident and we have to clean up before the resident sees it". I left and returned to the home a week later. The Officer in Charge was again unable to stop and talk to me. She told me that a resident had died and required "laying out", two double incontinents had soiled themselves and were in the process of being cleaned up and a psychiatric case had gone "beserk". I eventually did get to interview her and her first words were "You know Mr. Taylor people have absolutely no conception of the type of residents we get in these homes these days. They are so frail, confused and often incontinent we have no chance; we seem to be spending most of our time cleaning, nursing and toileting residents. All the activities we used to have regularly can't be done, every time we organize some sort of activity something happens with a resident or two and we have to postpone it. We don't seem to be able to get started again.[57]

From conversations with students on current courses, I have come to the conclusion that they are being pressured into finding something for residents to do between every meal and instructions appear to be geared to ambulant and mentally alert aged. There seems to be little or no definition of confusion and equally important, what can be done about it. Course tutors emphasize individuality and it is right that they should do so, yet they also make blanket statements regarding the general approach to care of the aged. [57:58]

One student said to me "I get worried as the tutors seem to advocate "jump in" and don't teach you to think of the consequences of any action you are about to take. Old people can be treated as adults on admission yet will find themselves playing childlike games as part of the 'motivation'. Staff often find that some handicrafts make their fingers sore and there is no possibility of the old people being able to engage in the activity for the same reason, or due to poor eyesight.

One home I know of has a very good relationship with the surrounding community. It is quite common for people to visit with the intention of involving the residents in some sort of activity. One of these people is a woman of 68, who goes to play cards with the residents and out of a total of 44, only two show any interest. The rest make it very plain to her that they do not wish to do anything, other than watch T.V. The Deputy of the home remarked "Staff lash themselves into a frenzy trying to get residents to join in games etc. and we are lucky if we get three. We played some records one night, the Officer in Charge and I danced with our wives and tried to coax the residents who were able to join in and all we got was you dance with your wives and we'll watch". Tutors tell residential workers that residents should be encouraged to make their own beds or even empty their commodes. Many do, but how does an old man or woman, who can only walk with the aid of a zimmer stand up to make their own bed? Many are unable to empty their commodes for the same reason and those that try invariably slop the contents onto the floor. I know an old man who has a catheter, he empties it himself, over the house plants! In the home I have just mentioned, only three make any attempt to make their own beds.

One student told me she had sat through a lecture where the tutor had spent the time telling them what residents should do. She said she sat and thought about each resident in her home and could not think of one who was capable of doing what the tutor had suggested. As she said "Tutors and many others think residents are all nice grandfathers and grandmothers, they visit a home for an hour during one afternoon and base their judgment on so short an acquaintance. They should visit when we are getting residents up or putting them to bed". This same woman related the following story to me. "I went on a course at the local hospital to learn methods of lifting residents. In our home, we had a very big lady, who was paralyzed down one side. We just could not lift her without assistance. She would go rigid or completely slack, depending on her mood. She would also switch from laughing to shouting in the space of seconds. While on this course, I asked advice about lifting this particular resident and the nurse who was instructing us got a very slight young woman to lie down and demonstrated the technique. I tried to tell her that the resident I was talking about weighed about three times that of her subject and tried to explain the other difficulties. All she said was, 'I think she is having you on my dear".[59]

I know a young man who was on a course and he said all the students became heartily fed up being told what to do with residents who are so confused and frail that 90% of them were unable to move without assistance. Eventually, they told the Course Tutors that they had no idea what they were talking about and they (the students) were dealing with practicalities and not theory and challenged the tutors to go and work in a home for the aged. One young woman accepted the challenge and it was arranged for her to work in a home for six weeks. She agreed to try every job in the home, start as a domestic, go on to Care Attendant them work with the Officer in Charge. Whatever the Officer in Charge did, she wanted to be there. If there was a call during the night she wanted to be called and in fact, she wanted to be the Officer in Charge's shadow. She lasted ten days!! She returned to the students and confessed she could not understand how they managed to do their jobs. She also expressed doubts about her knowledge of residential work and her ability to function as a tutor on the course. She must have found some way of salving her conscience as she is still tutoring and I will give her two out ten for trying.

Students are told they should sit with a dying resident. There are differences in all homes. Some may be able to do this, others may not and in any case, it depends again on having a full staff and, let us be honest, it is not a pleasant task. Very few relatives will do it though I have known some take turns and sit with a dying parent. Staff usually have to keep popping in as they go about their jobs. I have heard tutors say that residents should be allowed to grieve for one who has died, also that staff should grieve. If staff allowed themselves to grieve every time a resident died, they would spend most of their time dressed in "sackcloth and ashes". Of course, staff feel some sorrow when a resident dies, but they cannot let it continually affect their lives otherwise they would all finish up psychiatric cases. As for resident's attitudes to one of their number dying, the following incident should serve to illustrate a point.[60:61]

I was in a home with a vestibule come lounge. There were about 12 residents sitting there and four of them were playing cards. A resident had died during the previous night and the undertaker had called to take the body away and had to take the coffin past the residents. The Deputy Officer in Charge went to them and asked if they wanted to go to one of the other lounges as they were bringing Mrs.... through now, but one of the card players replied "No lad, never mind about us, just you carry on". He then turned to one of the other and said "It's your deal". The coffin was brought through and none took any notice. I did hear they all subscribed to a wreath.[60:61]

Staff I have spoken to say that most old people seem very philosophical about death. There are a few who seem to 'fight it' when the end is near but they are in the minority and those who are left seem to detach themselves very quickly and will think nothing of asking the same day a resident has left if they can have the vacant room or sit in a vacant place in the dining room. Staff tell me that when a resident has died, they rarely hear his/her name mentioned again. [60:61]

Back to motivation and I would like to pose a question. If as we are constantly being told, staff spend all their time talking to residents, who is going to do the other work.

The staff of an adapted home for 28 residents had all attended a series of lectures and taking the tutors suggestions to heart, they asked the Officer in Charge if they could put them into practice. Being rather forward looking, she agreed. The first thing the staff decided to do was take some of the residents to the Public House, about 200 yards from the main door of the home. They have not repeated the experiment. Two of the residents had to be carried back and another developed knee trouble and has had to have a zimmer ever since. Before someone says, "They should have used wheelchairs" let me point out that in this particular home there is no room for them and only ambulant residents are supposed to be admitted. The Officer in Charge remarked to me after relating this story "Perhaps staff will listen to what I say in future".

A number of old people do help with tasks about the home but a great many succumb to group pressure. A new resident may wish to help with the washing up, setting tables, dusting etc. and will be told by the rest, "If you do it we'll all have to and the next thing we'll be spending all day working, so stop it". I went on a routine visit to one of the homes I am responsible for. I chatted for a while with the residents, the great majority of whom have made it quite clear to staff and to me that they have no intention of doing anything, even making small articles for fund raising activities. In one of the lounges I noticed a lady I had not see before and as I left the lounge, she followed me out and stopped me in the hall. She asked who I was and what position I held. When I told her she said "Have the staff any right to make me set the tables?" I told her that I was sure staff were not making her do anything and tried to explain that even such a small task would help to keep her mobile and that if she sat in a chair all day she would very soon reach the point when she would not be able to move. I spoke to the Officer in Charge about the incident an she told me the old lady had been with them a week and had offered to help at the tables. She (the Officer in Charge) was delighted as she thought it might be the start of a breakthrough. After our talk, she realized that the old lady was looking for excuse to stop helping and this was her way of doing it.

I am not sure if the following has any significance, but it is worthy of your observation.

I have found that most of the old people in homes who do help themselves and keep busy in one way or another, have suffered some major affliction early in their lives and have had to come terms with it and seem grateful for the fact that they can do anything at all. There are quite a number I know, some unfortunately have died, who perform tasks that far more able bodied would not entertain. There is one old lady who is confined to a battery operated wheelchair. She collects the day care money keeps the records, types letters for the Officer in Charge, writes Pam Ayres type poetry, corresponds all over the world and goes out of her way to welcome new residents. A man who has been blind since he was a child types all the Officer's letters organizes and types the menu, also he occupies his time with handicrafts. There are double amputees, a man and a woman, both confined to wheelchairs. The man makes dozens of articles for sale at fund raising events; the woman spends most of her time painting in oils. She admits she is not very good at it but she keeps going. One lady, who is now dead, was confined to a wheelchair, physically handicapped, her body terribly twisted, yet she always had something to do, usually making soft toys or knitting and it always amazed me how she managed. Another lady, also in a wheelchair, was a Doctor of Psychology and many a pleasant talk I had with her. She was a sort of unofficial "enabler". If any of residents or all of them wanted anything, they went to her first and she spoke to the Officer in Charge.

These are just a few of the people I know, or have known, who made some effort on their own behalf and here also is a list of residents in a home administered by the R.N.I.D. and the duties they have adopted.

Woman 61 Schizophrenia	Collects washing after it has been done and gets it dried either outside or in the cellars. Brings the dry clothes to be ironed. Does shopping for anyone who wants things but needs watching or she will get their money mixed up with her own - always to her own advantage.
Man 75 Bad Heart.	Butters bread and gets things ready for the cook. Prepares vegetables and generally helps around kitchen.

Man 62 Deformed Spine	Helps with the tea time bread and butter. Sweeps the dining room floor after each meal and once a week mops and polishes the dining room floor. Walks the dog.
Woman 59 Retarded.	Does some of the ironing and serves the residents at meal times. If anyone is in bed, she takes their trays up.
Woman 56 Retarded	Does ironing not done by previous lady. Staircases to both floors are swept and dusted every morning and the top floor landing.
Woman 84	Puts away all clean linen both from laundry and that done in the home. Puts out sugar, milk, dishes, cake etc. and lays the tables for all meals. Helps to serve if everyone busy.
Man 72.	Keeps the back yard and shed tidy. Greengroceries are kept in back shed. He puts them all away in their boxes when they arrive. Does all Cook's washing up.
Man 93 Bad heart.	Does all washing up after residents meals, helped by three others.
Woman 84 Spastic.	Does all washing up after residents meals helped by three others. Sorts out dirty linen and puts what does not go to the laundry in the sluice room for washing. She folds and counts laundry for staff to check
Woman 62 Spastic	Cleans all wash basins in the residents bedrooms and the three bathrooms wash basins every day. Dusts first floor corridors.
Man 73 Retarded	Is fanatical about the big lounge, hall and small lounge. He dusts, polishes, vacs, waters plants etc. everyday. Once a week he cleans the ground floor windows inside and out and keeps the small garden at the front of the house and a lawn at the side of the house generally tidy

Woman 82+ Epileptic	Puts out all the clean sheets and pillow slips, hand towels, bath towels and face cloths and collects dirty ones for others.
Woman 64. Deaf- Deaf Blind TB Hip. One leg 3" shorter.	Does early morning tea at 6 a.m. Washes up and puts crockery away. Uses Braille typewriter, writes letters for other residents, corresponds with people all over the world. Best way to describe her is Social Worker to all other residents.
	The men have taken responsibility for securing the doors and windows at dusk. Seeing that all electrical equipment is unplugged and switched off at night. All ready to be checked by staff on late duty.

These people besides having the afflictions shown are all deaf and always have been.

As I see it, Residential Workers have one of two alternatives. They can either make old people do something, or encourage them. The former is unacceptable, therefore the latter only is left open to them. So the Residential Workers, if they have done all they can to encourage participation on the part of an old person without success, then in spite of what people say, they have to learn to settle for what they can get. If only 4 or 5 out of 40 residents are prepared to involve themselves in an activity or the running of the home, then any worker who frets and worries over those who do not, is heading for health problems.

Taken For A Ride- Michael Meacher

(57) All these things the matrons encourage, even to the extent of allowing their charges to take mild risks, which they felt were to be preferred to the frustration and hopelessness produced by constantly checking and forbidding them. Both set great store on the personal appearance of the old ladies, agreeing that feminine vanity was a valuable aid in maintaining self-respect. Nice clothes were encouraged and soft, becoming colours preferred to black and slate- grey. There were regular visits to the hairdresser, with the full flattering routine of a cup of tea and biscuits under the drier and picture magazines to look at. One of the Homes arranged sessions for removing facial hair for those who needed it. The underlying idea is that a normal appearance, normal surroundings and, as far as possible, a normal routine, are aids to normal behaviour (Roberts, 1961. pp 14-15)

(58) The widely experienced matrons of two homes caring exclusively for the mentally confused were virtually unanimous on general principles when they were consulted... There is general agreement that one of the best insurances against a restless night is a reasonably active and interesting day.... A daily walk, or mild pottering in the garden if an old lady is physically up to it, helps to work off their energy. The homes have discovered that even people who are rather noticeably astray can enjoy doing handwork of various kinds and produce quite creditable specimens, but few of them are capable of persevering at this kind of activity unless they are in a group with somebody to help and encourage them. 'Handwork' is a term that can be used widely. It can imply knitting blanket- squares or making felt rabbits; equally it may mean unravelling a pile of wool for an old lady who would otherwise be worrying her scarf or her bedcover to bits.

(59) When one particularly obese lady found herself embedded in the bath on one occasion the matron told me that she had been obliged to call in her husband to heave her out by force majeure.

Residential work with the Elderly- C. Paul Brearley

(56) An important element in the development of services for the older people is that of attitudes held by the community in general terms to 'old people', as well as the attitudes of professionals involved with the elderly, and the attitudes of the elderly themselves to their needs, to being old, and to the kind of care that is provided for them.

(60) Loss of all kinds associated with a subsequent period of adjustment or grieving. Grief is not only linked with loss of a person but can also relate to loss of a part of the self, or of good health, or of a house or possessions. It is to be expected then, that older people entering a home or hospital will require a period of grieving which may take several forms. It is possible to describe common elements of the grieving process. In the first few days a feeling of emptiness, numbness and disbelief is common in which denial is a common feature. After this a period of grief, despair and emptiness follows in which episodes of physical distress alternate with apathy and disinterest. Sometimes anger, relief or guilt are felt. Appropriate grieving will normally require outlets of expression; if these are not available pathological reactions - chronic grief may occur with excessive guilt, bitterness, anger or anxiety in evidence and occasionally hallucinations, delusions and physical reactions.

(61) The great majority of old people who live in an institutional setting will also die there. Death and dying are a common part of life in care and different establishments find different ways of handling this. Family and individual dignity should be respected in the way death and burial arrangements are handled. In residential care the stress is perhaps more to be placed on death then on the process of dying; residents either experience a brief terminal phase or they are admitted to hospital for longer term care. Most elderly residents will feel a need to talk about death at some time and to review their feelings about the approach of death. Some will say that they are ready for death, that they feel that they have lived a good and useful life and they are 'ready to go'. 'I wish

he'd come and take me' is a not uncommon comment and sometimes this kind of reaction may seem quite realistic. It may, however, be that this is a depressive form of reaction, and that what seems like a calm acceptance of the reality, may be apathetic depression.

Death in most hospitals and some residential homes is coped with in ritualized, standardised ways. Sometimes a more significant member of the communal group dies and leaves a major gap and the group must go through a period of grieving for their joint loss. The worker should be able to help them in their grieving and encourage them to see the loss in a realistic context.

Chapter 11

I have seen many people leave the work and having spoken to them regarding their reasons, I have come to the conclusion that the majority felt they could not do what they thought was expected of them. They admitted they had tried but were of the opinion that they were failures and.it is wrong for anyone to imply that staff are not doing their job properly if they do not get all the old people in their care to adopt some sort of regular activity. I put this to a retired Director of Social Services and he said, "If I live until I am 85, I don't bloody well want to be motivated. I'll please myself and if I want to doze in a chair after lunch, then I intend to do so". [62]

There was an old lady in a home; she had been blind for about two years. I discovered this was due to her having nursed a child who, it was found after, had German measles. Shortly after this incident, the old lady was found to have shingles and this affected her eyesight. She was admitted to hospital for treatment and before this was complete, she discharged herself. As her sight got worse and she could no longer manage, she was admitted to Part 111. She continued to refuse treatment and eventually lost her sight altogether. The officer in charge had spoken to the Consultant who had treated her and had been told that had the old lady continued with the treatment, she would have regained her sight. Physically and mentally, this lady was well and could have been quite active but she refused even to move without assistance. It so happened that the Officer in Charge had worked with the blind and knew how capable they were after proper training. Thinking to do the lady a service, she called in a Social Worker for the blind to teach the lady how to move around unaided. The lady refused to have anything to do with the Social Worker and said, "it's only because you don't want to be bothered with me. This is what I get for helping a person. I'm a poor blind old woman. I came in here to be looked after but you don't want to do it". This went on for months with the resident bewailing her fate daily and accusing staff of ignoring her. Eventually, the staff did a small survey on her and found that she had the undivided attention of member of staff on no less then 17 occasions during the waking hours. The lady, although physically capable, had to be led to the toilet, the dining room, bedroom, and lounges and even had to be dressed, as she could not dress herself. She was unable to read and relied on others to do it for her and she could not watch T.V. and while other residents were watching, she would switch on her radio and disrupt the whole lounge. When the inevitable happened, she would complain, "you can all see but you deny me my only bit of pleasure". Eventually, staff had to be quite hard with her for the sake of the others and sit her in the hall where she could have her radio all to herself.[62]

In the same home was a woman who was the youngest of them all by a long way. She had been in Part 111 twice. The first time she had been admitted because she was found in bed soaked in urine and soiled with faeces. She was kept in the home for a few months rehabilitation and her house was cleaned up for her. After she had been discharged for a few weeks, the Field Worker called and found her in the same state as before. She was readmitted to Part 111 and it was decided to keep her as all involved were of the opinion she would continue to behave in the same way if she were to go out. She was in the home for several years and would do nothing for herself or any of the others. She hardly moved from her chair even to go out in the summer and she smoked like a chimney. She also became very obese. A new Officer in Charge was appointed to the home and spoke to the doctor about the resident. He recommended a strict diet and some activity. The Officer in Charge, whilst agreeing with the doctor, could not give the resident the kind of work she needed. The doctor suggested she start by helping with the washing up and setting tables and he would tell her so and, being a man of his word, did. It was not long before the Officer had to start replacing crockery. The resident only broke a few at a time but she was consistent. There was almost a complete renewal of crockery over a few months. The resident was taken out of the kitchen and given a duster but staff soon found that ornaments, plant pots and glass fronted cabinets are more expensive than cups and saucers. The Officer in Charge was heard to remark "god knows what she would do with a bucket of water and a mop". After trying all they could think of, the staff admitted defeat. As for the diet, they got nowhere as she got other residents and visitors to bring food in to her and she ate it secretly.[62]

Some old people will go to great lengths to impress upon staff the fact that they <u>expect everything</u> to be done for them. There was an old man of 80+ who was admitted to a part 111 home, quite active and mentally alert. A home adviser received a complaint from him about his treatment in the home. When the Homes Adviser spoke to the old man, he found his complaint was only that the Officer in Charge would not shave him. The Officer told the old man he was perfectly capable of shaving himself and that he, the Officer in Charge, had no intention of waiting on him hand and foot. The old man started being difficult and unco-operative and demanded to be moved to another home – he got his wish. Shortly after the move, he made his way to the office, which was three miles from the home, using a zimmer to help him walk the distance. He asked to see the Director but was again seen by the Homes Advisor and this time his complaint was that staff would not get him a box of matches. He did not have another suit to put on and had no clean shirts. It transpired he had asked a member of staff who was going off duty to get him a box of matches and she had brought them with her the next day when she returned. She admitted quite frankly, she was not inclined to drop everything she was doing and run around to suit him. She also pointed out that the shop was only 50 yards from the door. The Officer in Charge also said the old man deliberately wrenched the buttons of his suits and would also tear his shirts and it was with utmost difficulty that staff managed to get him a change of clothes to wear. The Homes Advisor was shown the old man's wardrobe. In it were two perfectly good suits with buttons missing. The Officer in Charge said they had stopped putting clean shirts and underwear in the chest of drawers and kept them out of the old man's way until he was ready to change. The Officer in Charge said the old man was still demanding to be shaved and asked how he (the old man) could walk 3 miles to the office and would not walk 50 yards to the shop. The old man mumbled a bit and said staff were paid to look after him and his pension book was taken from him to pay them. He finished by demanding to be moved to another home. Again he was moved and the last I heard was that the third home were having the same problems with him.[62] Isn't it surprising that if a child or resident in a home asks to be moved, they will get their move in a reasonably short time but if staff ask for someone to be moved they will be told it cannot be done and all sorts of excuses will be trotted out to justify this reluctance.

An old man of 70+ was admitted to a part 111 home and from the first day, he made it apparent that he had no intention of doing a thing, also he proved to be totally unco-operative and abused staff continually. When there were no staff about he would abuse and insult the other residents. After a week in the home his daughter, a woman in her early forties, went to visit him and he started to abuse her. The Officer in Charge was a witness to this and when the daughter was about to leave called her into the office. The Officer in Charge asked the daughter if she could throw any light on the old man's behaviour and the daughter gave the following information. Her father had treated her and her mother like drudges. Her mother, now dead, had led a miserable life and for the sake of peace had pandered to his every whim. When her mother had died, her father had turned his attention to her. She had held down a full time job to support them both and as he would not lift a finger, she had all the housework, shopping, washing etc. to do herself. She had never been able to have a male friend home as her father drove them away. If she tried to meet anyone away from the house her father followed her and abused them. She told the Officer in Charge she had met a man who wanted to marry her and she felt she deserved some happiness in life and that she had got her father in the home out of sheer desperation. She said she had just told him she had become engaged and that was why he was abusing her. He had accused her of "fornicating and bloody well carrying on with men behind his back and he wasn't staying in this so and so prison just so she could sleep with a man". She told the Officer in Charge that she would be moving to another address so her father could not find her and would leave it with the Officer in Charge only on the solemn promise that the father would not be told and that if he needed anything they were to let her know and she would see that he got it. The Officer in Charge promised that the old man would not get to know where his daughter had gone and wished the lady every happiness. All the time the man was in the home the daughter telephoned three times a week to ask about him but would not visit. After his daughter's visit, the man became worse, so bad that other residents ostracised him completely and asked the Officer in Charge to get him moved. They were told this would not be fair, as they would only be pushing their problems on to someone else. One member of staff remarked, "no wonder his wife died, she was probably glad to go, he is a wicked old swine". The man proceeded to make life intolerable for all around him. He asked the Officer in Charge if she knew where his daughter was and was told, "Yes, but that he was not getting the address". He called the Officer in Charge "a bloody old cow" and went and put a coat on and went out. The police brought him back some hours later. He had gone to his old address and found the house empty. The police had found him wandering the streets and when they had stopped him he had abused them but had told them where he had come from. This became quite a habit and as the police got to know him, they just returned him to the home each time they saw him. Staff went to considerable trouble to try and help him to settle. The Officer in Charge had several talks with him and told him he might as well content himself, as his daughter was married and he was not going to get the opportunity to break it up. He started on something of a hunger strike. Nothing the staff did for him suited him and always met with abuse. The Officer in Charge bought a particular delicacy for him which he had said he liked. The first time it was served to him he ate it and the next day when the evening meal was announced, he remained seated in the lounge. The Officer in Charge went to see him and he said he wanted nothing to eat. The Officer in Charge told him she had got some more of the food he liked and asked him to go to the dining room. His reply was "it's too bloody far". The dining room was 20 yards from him. The next ploy on the part of this man was refusal to go to the toilet, so staff had to clean and change him regularly. Staff became heartily sick of him and when he died none showed any distress. His daughter made a donation to the home and thanked the staff for putting up with him for so long.[46]

An old lady in a home never missed an opportunity to tell staff that she was paying their wages and expected them to wait on her. She would walk round the home and point out any work she deemed to have been missed. Every morning, she would pull all the bedclothes off her bed and throw them on the floor. She told staff they would not just pull the blankets up, she would see to it that they would have to make her bed from 'scratch'.

A diabetic old lady was admitted to a home from hospital. Her legs were hard and swollen and on admission, she weighed 12 and a half stones. With careful diet, she lost weight and her legs returned to normal. She insisted she was not a diabetic and that staff were starving her, which caused a number of arguments. She demanded to be washed, dressed, undressed and put to bed. Eventually, staff became a bit fed up with her and the Officer in Charge told her she was perfectly capable of helping herself and that staff would no longer wait upon her. This brought forth accusations of cruelty. The Officer in Charge said to her, "you can call me what you like and report me to who you like but you are going to help yourself!!" after some weeks, the old lady got the message and started to make an effort on her own behalf. [62]

In the same home there is an old lady with angina and if she does not want to do anything, or is not getting the attention she wants, she will have a heart attack. She usually does this when she thinks it is her turn for a bath. She objects to soap and water. Alternatively, she will be ill, staff have to settle for strip washing her and staff say if they peep around the door after she has gone to bed, she will have tipped the drawers out and will be busy tidying them.

In contrast, another lady in another home was said to have a very bad heart and was not to do anything for herself. She slept in a multiple bedroom. A relative took her to a party and returned her a 4.00a.m. The night staff had to call the Officer in Charge to assist her in getting her to bed and in the process all the other residents were awakened. The Officer in Charge mentioned the incident to the doctor who was attending the resident and he said, "Report her, get her moved". What good reporting her or getting her moved would have done goodness knows. When the Officer in Charge pointed this out to the doctor he replied, "I wouldn't put up with it" and he had some hard words to say to the old lady about her "bad heart".

An old man of 79 suffered from urine retention and a heart condition. He continually abused staff and refused to take his medication when they asked him, so the most they could do was leave his with him as he said "it is none of your bloody business when I take my tablets". This went on for several weeks until one night at about 10 o'clock the member of staff on duty noticed he was obviously not well. The Officer in Charge was called who, in turn, called the doctor. When the doctor arrived, staff showed him all the tablets the resident had not taken and the doctor gave him an injection and it was 1.00a.m. Before they could leave him.

There was a similar case in another home involving an old lady of 70+. The doctor had prescribed some drugs for her condition. Staff gave her the prescribed number of tablets at the correct time and to all intents she was taking them. The resident grew progressively worse and the doctor changed her tablets on several occasions. Both he and staff were at a loss to understand the deterioration in her condition. The reason came to light by chance. The resident, due to her condition, reached the stage where she had to stay in bed. A member of staff went to tidy her wardrobe and in the process found a handbag. In the handbag were 450 assorted tablets, which she was supposed to have taken. The condition of the tablets indicated that they had been in her mouth. Staff came to the conclusion that when had given her the tablets she had put them in her mouth and spat them out when they had turned their backs. Had she not kept them, she would very likely have died and no-one would have been any the wiser. When the doctor next visited and was told, he was furious and asked to be left alone with the resident. It is not known what he said to her but she took her tablets from then on and her condition improved very rapidly.

An old man was admitted to a home from the community. He was shown to his room by the Deputy Officer in Charge, who helped him unpack his belongings. In the process of doing this, he remarked on the absence of a razor and the old man said, "I was told not to bring one as staff would shave me". The authority responsible for the home had spent quite a lot of the money at the Officer in Charge's request to have all the mirrors and washbasins in the rooms lowered, in order that the residents could do more for themselves.

Many staff are becoming increasingly concerned at the number of psychiatric cases currently being placed in Part 111 homes.

One home had four women residents who had very bad hearts and because of this, as you will no doubt appreciate, had to be treated very carefully. The Officer in Charge accepted a "swap" from the hospital. She did not go to hospital to assess the new resident and when I asked her why, she said, "I was given no choice, I was told they only had the one and if I didn't take her there wouldn't be a bed for my sick resident. I was also told she had been in a psychiatric ward but that she had been stabilised and was alright". The new resident was admitted and for 24 hours she was fine. The second evening, the Officer in Charge was going around the lounge giving out the tablets. When she went to the new resident the tray was snatched from her and thrown across the room. The resident struck out at her with a walking stick and then threw the walking stick at another resident and started attacking others in the lounge. The Officer in Charge telephoned the hospital and asked why they had misled her and also told them they could not cope with the woman and that if she attacked any of those with bad hearts, the shock would kill. Believe it or not, the hospital member of staff replied, "That is just your hard luck". Eventually, the resident was moved but not until the Officer in Charge threatened them with a written report to the Area Health Officer.[65]

A 91-year-old woman, a psychiatric case, nearly succeeded in strangling a lady in for a day care because she said the day care was wearing her coat. The same woman will attack other residents with her walking stick if they wear a white cardigan, which she says is hers.

Some people may say that a person of that age does not have much strength but residential staff know only too well that old people are surprisingly strong when the mood takes them. In the above case, it took two members of staff to break her grip. Psychiatrists will tell homes that such cases are not dangerous to them. I question such inept comments – they may not be a danger to staff but they are a great danger to frail residents. As I have already said, knowledge of Part 111 homes is abysmal. As one Officer in Charge said to me, "These people conveniently forget that mental nursing is a specialised field of which we have no knowledge and it is totally unreasonable to expect us to cater for this on top of everything else. We are becoming nothing less then dumping grounds".

Taken for a ride – Michael Meacher

Sporadically in the separatist homes authoritarianism spilled over and into actual staff violence. Such eruptions, even if infrequent, are perhaps inevitable in residential establishments for the elderly where staffing schedules are typified by worker shortage and hence excessive work loads, long hours of duty and the need to deal with an unusually high incidence of disturbed behaviour. Furthermore the built-in tendency towards residents' long-term physical and mental deterioration undermines the prestige of the work and thus exacerbates recruitment and turnover problems. Certainly these hazards have received widespread adverse publicity from the exposures of recent reports.

(65) In one case when two women quarrelled and one slapped the other's face, the latter complainted to her son who immediately tried to have his mother's assailant removed by the police. Again, when a woman gruffly told her bedroom companion to pull herself together, the latter's daughter remonstrated with the matron because her mother was arthritic and in no fit condition, and sought the complainant's transfer to another bedroom. And another resident's children lodged a protest on the grounds that their mother had to sit next to an incontinent and disoriented neighbour, though this was the sole instance discovered of such a complaint. Both these protégées were rational. Interestingly enough, in view of the former example, when a severely confused resident was struck in similar circumstances, no protest was forthcoming from the family.

Residential Work with the Elderly – C. Paul Brearly

(62) Role-deprivation is a consequence of growing old; entry to an old people's home or hospital will involve role-loss. Those who go into an enclosed environment leave behind them many active roles; they may cease being tenants, householders or neighbours, they stop being people who pay the milkman or who hold their own rent book and collect their own pension. The loss of all these roles, and the reciprocal

relationship that they imply at a time of other major life changes, adds up to considerable personal deprivation. It is vital that older people in institutions are given the opportunity to regain self-esteem and to rebuild their self-concept. One way of helping them to do this will be the simple recognition, by staff, of their right to respect, and of their difference from other residents.

Residential Care Reviewed P.S.S.C. 1977

Most elderly people admitted to hospital are discharged within three months. It is therefore suggested that where the resident of an old people's Home is admitted to hospital his or her place in the Home should be retained for approximately three months, unless advice from the consultant in charge of the case indicates that a much longer period in hospital is unavoidable. In order to make the best use of residential provision, places temporarily unoccupied as a result of hospital admissions should be added to the stock of places available for short-stay residential care, full consideration being given to safeguarding the personal property, furniture and belongings of the resident whose room is being used. Policy on the retention of places should be sufficiently flexible to allow sympathetic consideration of each case on its merits, and where doubt about a possible discharge exists, the place should be retained.

Volunteers. It is in no way to detract from the importance of adequate and qualified staffing in homes to recognise the additional value of using voluntary workers. The volunteer can also provide time, personal help, additional skills, and activities that the staff cannot always make available; he/she can reduce the risk of institutionalisation and extend the range of opportunities, interests and relationships open to residents; far more can be done on the same budget with his/her help than without. Yet he/she is often regarded with suspicion, and it is sometimes said that volunteers can be more of a hindrance than a help.

Special consideration needs to be given to the care of those who are very frail and infirm. Because of the increase in number of the very elderly relative to the population as a whole, there is growing pressure on homes to accept people who require a higher degree of physical and nursing care than the home is intended to provide. This is damaging to the residents and limiting for the potential of residential care. Either the care provided by homes should be reconsidered and their objectives changed to embrace the very frail or handicapped, or closer collaboration should be assured with the health service, in order that respective responsibilities can be properly exercised. Consultations should take place jointly between the social services and the health service on this matter; both at the level of the home in relation to local practices and as a matter of policy at local authority and area health authority level. If the very frail are to be the responsibility of local authorities, then some homes will require to be equipped with staff and facilities accordingly. It is misguided to place difficult demands upon homes and staff, as happens at the present time, without providing the resources to meet them. The result is an inability to give proper care either to the frail or to the capable residents.

Do staff understand how to deal with bereavement? When a resident dies do they keep the fact quiet, announce it publicly, tell other residents individually? Can they discuss the subject of death without embarrassment? Do they understand the need of people to be able to discuss death freely in fact? Do they know how to help a resident whose close friend has died, either within or without the home, or who has lost a relative? Do they have any counselling or help to enable them to do so? Is this a subject they are encouraged to discuss among themselves so that they can help each other?

Do staff receive help in dealing with terminal care? Are they nervous about discussing it and unsure how to treat the dying resident? Do they understand the philosophical approach old or handicapped people often have to death? Do they encourage relatives or other residents to help? Do they try to hush it up, and if so, have they considered the possible reactions of other residents when they considered the possible reactions of other residents when they realise own final illness may be hushed up in the same way? Do they appreciate that their own attitudes can inhibit those in their care from openly expressing essential mourning or fears about dying?

(77) 'Handicapped persons develop a feeling of isolation from the community in spite of frequent visits by members of the public... there should be more publicity about the feeling of isolation and need for more integration between disabled people and the community at large' (Resident and staff)

'Boredom and lethargy is quite a problem in a residential home. To be kept in touch with the world outside plus indoor activities arranged by the staff would help to stimulate them' (Staff)

'I would say the overcoming of boredom is an important part in the daily life of the resident in care... the probable majority of residents enter into care with practically everything done for them, having always been used to fending for themselves' (Relative)

Do staff give priority to seeing that residents are occupied or do they consider this of little importance? Do they look at the pattern of the day from the angle of the residents? Are residents free to choose what they do? Are they asked if they wish to undertake tasks in the home or to assist in some duties such as bed making? Do staff let residents know when help is needed by other residents, which they could give, such as shopping, letter writing, assistance with feeding or dressing?

Are residents encouraged to take exercise? Is the value of this in maintaining both health and independence realised? If residents take little exercise is it ever asked whether this is because they lack the reassurance of a companion on a walk? Are visitors encouraged to take walks with residents instead of only sitting to talk with them?

Residents cannot live full and interesting lives if all choice and responsibility is removed from them. It is the function of the staff to help residents to develop their potential not to stultify them by over-protection; to assist people to do things for themselves not to increase their dependence by doing everything for them. This can be difficult to carry out; it is often easier to do something for a resident rather than, apparently ruthlessly, leave him/her to struggle unaided. It can both satisfy better the instinctive that residents lose their skills and abilities if these are not utilised or never develop them if they are not required to do so. Both mental and physical determination often occurs after admission because of lack of need to do even simple tasks like dressing, bed making or cooking, or to apply the mind even to the simple of decisions, such as choosing a menu.

'It helps to get out to Old People's Clubs and to go on outings arranged by various organisations and to get a chance to talk to someone outside the home' (Resident)

'Company and not gifts of sweets and flowers would be welcome' (Staff)

'All they do is keep her clean, warm and fed. No stimulation (except television (?)) is offered and the old ladies just sit staring into space. If only they had to do exercise or sing to an accompaniment they would come to life occasionally – as it is they just wait to die – at least it's an escape from boredom' (Relative)

Chapter 12

I recently read the booklet "Management for Continence" written by Bob Brown and published by Age Concern and I have discussed it with Officers in Charge who have also read it. The general opinion of those I have talked to seems to be that while Bob Brown's recommendations are perfectly sound, their success depends on two major factors:- (1) a full staff to implement them and (2) a reasonable number of incontinent to cater for. I know of Officers in Charge who have tried to put the recommendations into practice, only to have them fall flat because staff have not turned into work. As one Officer in Charge remarked "What do I do with 28 residents, 10 of whom are incontinent, 4 doubly and only myself and one Case Assistant on duty?". I take Bob's point about the siting of toilets. Many of the more recently built homes do have toilets sited more sensibly but the problem of the confused and non-ambulant remains to exacerbate the situation. The confused resident is often unaware that they need to go to the toilet and by the time the non or less ambulant realise they need to go, it is too late and they cannot get there in time. The situation in adapted properties, as many will know, is much worse and I cannot see the authorities spending money to provide more or resiting existing toilets in these homes.[66:67]

One situation comes to mind. I was discussing this with a Residential Worker, a Deputy Officer in Charge who has the C.S.S. Certificate. He and his Officer in Charge had set out to implement Bob Brown's recommendations and had chosen just a few of their more incontinent residents. One was a man of 80+ who was also severely confused. Both agreed that using the toilet was a very private function, so that old man was charted and toileted as suggested but when they went to collect him again after a reasonable time and adjusted his clothes, he would defecate in his trousers and trail faeces around the home. Both admitted that after considerable effort over a fair period, they are no further forward.[66:67] This is only one of a number of cases, which have been related to me, and Officers in Charge say they are already becoming overwhelmed with paperwork. In consequence, they view anything, which increases this with a certain amount of suspicion. Also, administrators and a large section of the community fail to realise, or refuse to admit, that some old people will, and do, use incontinence as a weapon and any success we achieve or hope to, needs the co-operation of the client/resident – call them what you will. Far too many people, a large section of whom lay claim to 'professionalism' or knowledge of the needs of the aged go into homes and see adult human beings. They cannot grasp the fact that old people regress or behave like spoiled children and will use any ploy they consider suitable to gain their own way. When staff are faced with a resident of this type, there is little or nothing they can do about it. I know of staff who, having taken a resident to the toilet return for her and open the toilet door with their foot because the resident smears the walls and door handles with faeces. Staff admit that toileting this type of resident is a major operation, as they have to prepare themselves with cleaning materials before they start.[66:67] In another home, a resident goes to the toilet herself but wraps her faeces up in paper and throws it out of the window. So far there has been no complaints from passers by! Another resident wraps her faeces up in her stockings. Whatever the psychiatric explanation for this, they are of very little assistance to staff, as if they wish to ensure that the resident is kept clean and avoid causing offence to others, also avoid objectionable smells in the home, then they must watch the residents using the toilet and so it ceases to be a private function.

Many staff, though not happy about it, use incontinence pads not purely for expediency but for the peace of mind of the residents as, although the residents may be upset at the prospect of the incontinence pad, they are even more distressed if they soil their clothes and have to be bathed and changed and, as staff say, "We can cope with a reasonable amount of incontinence but couple that with confusion and lack of mobility and the situation because impossible".[91]

Can I now return to Age Concern and confusion in the aged. I saw part of an article on T.V. dealing with confusion. The man speaking was a professor who worked for Age Concern and while I am prepared to agree with him that confusion is a curable state. I was somewhat annoyed towards the end when he made a comment which made me realise he was talking about slight confusion. I began to think about his recommendations and the number of staff that would be required to implement them just for the mildly confused in homes I know.

I spoke to a lady I know who used to work for Age Concern and is now Officer in Charge of a Part 111 home. She had nothing but praise for Age Concern and the work they do. While she worked for them she had been involved with the confused and was happy to tell me of the success they enjoyed. I asked her what she thought of her chances of success in her present work and she said "Very little, I have neither the staff nor facilities". Now, you may think I am setting out to knock Age Concern. I assure you this is not my aim. I set out with the intention of writing about the practical problems, which Residential Workers are faced with every day.

One Deputy Officer in Charge saw the article mentioned above and that afternoon they took a group of residents to Blackpool illuminations. The next morning she thought she would try the professor's suggestions with a confused man who had been on the trip. He could not remember how he had enjoyed his afternoon and could not remember which afternoon until she reminded him. He then asked what had been so special about it. She told him where they had gone and what they had done. She told me she spent a little over an hour with this one resident and towards the end he vaguely remembered some lights but could not remember what kind. She left him for a few hours and then went back to try again and spend another one and a half hours with him, but said she got absolutely nowhere. He could not remember a thing. She said to me, "You know Mr. Taylor, I spent two and a half hours with that one resident and I have another 39 to be catered for and a third of those are confused, we just haven't the staff to spend so much time with each resident". She went on to say, "It's not only the number of staff we would need but the quality. Where are we going to find the type of people who could stand the strain of talking to and trying to motivate severely confused residents all day long?"

A young male deputy of a Part 111 home was doing a C.S.S. Course and as part of his studies, he was required to do a case study of a resident. In his home was an old lady who was supposed to be confused. The deputy chose this lady for his subject. As the information they had in the home about the lady was very sketchy and consisted of a few lines on a medical card he realised he would have to obtain a file relating to the past history. As the old lady had been in care for sometime, the deputy found the Field Worker who had originally admitted the lady had been gone for long time and there had been a succession of Field Workers over that period. It took the Deputy six weeks to trace the file. It was finally found in a box locked away in a cupboard. When he read through it, he realised the information it contained threw considerable light on the resident's supposed confusion. The possession of this information enabled him to embark on a positive treatment programme with the resident, which, in a very short time produced a dramatic improvement in her condition.

It is a very sad fact that the above case is all too common. Old people are placed in homes and the amount of social background information which staff receive would fill a postage stamp. It is obvious that in this case, the old lady was admitted to a home and forgotten. The case file had never been handed over with the case load to each successive field worker so, for quite some time the old lady did not have a Social Worker. In short, she was "dead" the day she was admitted. The area officer in this particular case is the type who resists passing on any information and pleads confidentiality, which implies that Residential Workers are incapable of treating social background information with the confidence it merits. This sort of situation is a sore point with the residential workers. They are expected to embark on a course of action in complete absence of knowledge or on someone else's views. I fail to see why, when a person is admitted to a home, the case file is not handed to the Officer in Charge and kept in the home. It would always be available and when the resident dies, it could then be locked away in a cupboard. This reluctance to pass on full information is not peculiar to old people, as many Residential Workers well know, but more of this later.

A young woman, third in charge of the home, was getting married. She was very kind to the residents and they all liked her. The Officer in Charge thought that since they were all so fond of her, they might like to contribute towards a wedding present. He went around the lounge to collect the money. Many displayed their regard for the young woman in their generosity, others gave 2p or 5p and in lounge was a resident said to be confused. When the Officer in Charge approached her, she asked what it was for. The Officer in Charge told her and she said, "I've never heard of her" and refused to contribute. A short time later the Officer in Charge had occasion to go into the same lounge and the same residents called him and said, "You know that's why I was sent in here ". The Officer in Charge said he didn't understand and the resident replied, "Because I can't remember". I leave it for you to think about.

So far, I have tried to keep the 'problems' that Residential Workers face separate but I am at the stage where I cannot keep everything in tidy little sections. If I could, then residential work would be shown to be as easy as winking. In this chapter, I have written about genuine and doubtful incontinence and confusion but there are number of things, some I have already quoted, which in themselves are a cause or an effect. Some of these are verbal and/or physical abuse and surprising though it may seem to some, residents sexuality. Also there are residents who just will not use the toilet, even when staff remind them or try to help.

There was an old man of 80+. He was deaf, partially sighted and hemiplegic. He had a calliper on one leg and walked with the aid of a stick. He was a sloppy eater and would not use a table napkin and, in consequence, his clothes were usually stained or smeared in food and although capable, he would not change them. He was too confused to move or allow staff to change him. Any attempt at help would result in him lashing out with walking stick and he would throw his stick at any other resident unwise enough to comment of his intractability.[69:91]

A man of 78 was admitted to a home. After a few weeks, staff reported to the Officer in Charge that he had become incontinent. This went on for some months and the Officer in Charge had a talk with staff about it. They maintained that the resident was sometimes doubly incontinent several times a day. The Officer in Charge was at a loss to understand, as he had no problems with the man. This particular Officer in Charge, when he related the story to me said, "You know how it is in residential work, Mr.Taylor I had a niggling in the back of my mind about this man, there was something about it which bothered me and I couldn't sort it out". The Officer in Charge started to make some enquiries into the man's past and found he had been something of a womaniser. It was then, as he put it "it clicked" – the man was only incontinent when the women were on duty. He took careful note over a couple of weeks. The man went to the toilet when he (the Officer in Charge) was on duty but staff reported incontinence when he was off. The Officer in Charge decided on a course of action, which meant putting himself to considerable trouble and inconvenience. He told staff that if the resident was incontinent and he himself was on the premises, they were to call him and he would do the bathing and changing. If he was going out anywhere, chemist, bank, office etc..., he would let them know how long he expected to be and they could then decide if they could leave the resident until he got back. The Officer in Charge told me "the old tomcat was getting sexual satisfaction from the woman cleaning him up but once he realised that I would be the only one to do it, it stopped. The resident thought he had my turns worked out but I've confused the issue so much, he's lost".[67:91]

I have talked to staff who are of the opinion that some residents, men and women, are deliberately incontinent and will make themselves sore, in order to get someone to touch their genitalia. As staff say, the resident has to be washed, dried and creamed to prevent chapping and they obtain sexual gratification in the process.[67:91]

There was a man of 88, whose wife virtually killed herself looking after him. While he was at home he would not accept any form of social help. The home help was told not to go to the house again, the doctor was discouraged from calling by the wife because of the trouble it caused her. Eventually, his wife became very ill through trying to cater for him and he was admitted to a Part 111 home. This home said he was confused and became violent when he did not get the attention he demanded. He was moved to another home and large doses of Largactil had to be used to control him. The doctor attending the home became quite concerned as the man would open his trousers in the lounge and play with himself. He would also lie naked on his bed and ask female staff "to stroke his balls". The doctor made some enquiries into the background of the case. He and the staff formed the opinion that the trouble was due to the fact that the man had been taken from a complete caring situation and that the transition was too much for him.

The Officer in Charge of the home had very worrying time with an old lady, who it was thought was haemorrhaging. This happened on a number of occasions and each time the doctor was called and each time no reason could be found. A thought occurred to the Officer in Charge and she told staff to watch the resident closely. The reasons soon came to light; the old lady was masturbating until she bled.

The husband of an Officer in Charge was going out of their flat one night and an old lady was coming out of the lift. The husband said, "Off to bed love". "Yes" said the old lady. I'll be along in ten minutes" said the husband and the old lady replied "By God lad, I wish you would!".

The staff of a home were trying to get a particularly difficult resident to bed. She was noted for being abusive and violent and was prone to very rapid swings of mood. The staff, having no success, called for help from the Deputy Officer in Charge. He helped them get her into bed and as he was leaving the bedroom the resident said to him "Hey you". The Deputy turned and the old lady pulled back the bedclothes and said, "There's a cunt here if you want to use it".

I know a home where there is a 70+ spinster. Staff are fully aware that she has more of the men then any other female resident. Staff say it is quite common to see a male resident in his underpants going to her room late at night or in the early hours of the morning. As the officer in charge remarked to me, "I doubt there will be many unwanted babies!!"

While I am the first to admit that old people are vulnerable, I would also remind you that staff are also and in fact they are very vulnerable and it is quite surprising the type of people who believe, without question, everything a severely confused resident tells them.

There was an 80-year-old lady in a home. She was very confused and, as there was no possibility of her returning home, her affairs had to be sorted out. For one reason or another, it had to be done by a Solicitor. The Solicitor arrived at the home and asked to see his client, he was shown to a private room and the old lady was brought to him. About two hours later, the Solicitor knocked on the office door and asked to speak to the Officer in Charge. He was in the middle of relating what the old lady had said to him when the Officer in Charge burst out laughing. The Solicitor was somewhat annoyed at the outburst and the Officer in Charge apologised and said, "I can't help it. What your client has told you is pure drivel, she is so confused she doesn't know if she is on this earth or fullers". The Officer in Charge then proceeded to enlighten the Solicitor as to the truth regarding his client. The Solicitor then tore up his notes, gave the Officer in Charge a legal document and said, "Just get her to sign this where it is indicated and I will do the rest". When this particular Officer in Charge related this story to me he said, laughing, "Mr. Taylor, you should have seen that chap's face, it was a picture".

There was a similar case related to me, only this time the "Star turn" was, of all things, a Psychiatrist. He had called at the home to see an old lady who had been referred to him. He did not see the Officer in Charge before seeing his client. After a fairly lengthy session, he went to the office to discuss his findings with the Officer in Charge. After he had been talking a short time the Officer in Charge said, "Do you realise that old woman is thoroughly confused and doesn't know what she is saying, in fact she will agree with anything anyone says to her? You had better let me see your notes. He went over to them, took out his pen and started crossing out. When he finished, there were none of the written comments untouched. The Psychiatrist sheepishly bid him good day and left. The Officer in Charge said to me "Mr. Taylor, wouldn't you think a man in his position would have the sense to speak to senior staff first and get some background information". They never saw that Psychiatrist again.

There was a man of 85 in a home. In his younger days, he had been a great rugby player. He was very confused and was always telling residents and staff about how much 'stick' he had taken in the ruck and how much he had given. He was coming out of the toilet one day, his shirt hanging out and his trousers were undone when the Officer in Charge saw him and took him into the washroom adjacent to the toilet at the same time saying "you can't wander around the home like that Mr...". Fortunately for the Officer in Charge there was another man who was mentally alert in the washroom at the same time. The Officer in Charge tucked the old man's shirt in and fastened his trousers, then took him back to the lounge. As soon as the Officer in Charge left, the old man started to tell the other residents, "that big chap (the Officer in Charge) just had me in a room and has really given me some stick". He went on in this vein for some time and some of the residents obviously believed him, as they indicated their intention of reporting the matter to the office. At this point, the second man entered the room and said after hearing the remarks, "You bloody liar, he did nothing of the sort" and he then told the other residents what had really happened. The same confused man told his son that one of the male staff was putting him through it and kept getting hold of "his balls". The son related this to the Officer in Charge, who questioned the staff member who was horrified at the suggestion. He did say that he occasionally would pinch the old man's bottom when he passes him and make some sort of rugby remark (he was also a rugby player). The Officer in Charge gave the staff member a talk on vulnerability and confusion.

A 90-year-old resident was in bed ill. She was not regarded as confused. The Officer in Charge saw to it that she was visited regularly. Whenever she was asked if she wanted anything she said, "No everything is alright, I have all I need". After a few days, she got up. When she went into the lounge she told them she had only got up because they (the staff) had left her alone and no one had been in to see her.

In the same home, another woman resident was not too well and had elected to stay in her room. The Officer in Charge sent a new young staff member to her with a cup of tea. The following day the resident was in the lounge and the Officer in Charge asked how she felt. "I'm alright" said the resident "but that

Care Assistant is a thief, she's stolen my purse". The Care Assistant heard the accusation and protested her innocence. The resident continued to accuse her of stealing and eventually reduced the Care Assistant tears. The resident had mislaid it. She did not apologise to the Care Assistant for the distress she had caused her.

There was an old lady in a home who was severely confused, though she had an excellent appetite and ate everything staff put before her. When she had finished she meals, she would take food from the others on her table and would tell her relatives that staff were starving her and this caused continual problems. For the sake of peace at meal times staff took to ensuring that the resident always had a piece of bread on her plate, at least whilst others were at the table eating. Staff even had to take her serviette away from her because she kept dipping it in her tea and trying to eat it.

I have only related four cases but when such incidents are related to other residents and embellished in the telling, then told to relatives or visitors, residential Staff are regarded as monsters because most people believe these stories and make no efforts to check their authenticity before telephoning the office and alleging malpractice.

There are many other ways residents use to gain attention and in doing so give outsiders a totally wrong impression of residential homes.

An old man who was being assisted with a change of suit for his usual visit to the local. He was very concerned about his money, which was in his suit he had taken off. The staff emptied the pockets of crumpled notes which when they were straightened out and counted amounted to more than £30. The resident was on to a good thing when he went to the Public House, he would be welcomed sympathetically and not allowed to buy his own drinks or even encouraged to because "he was a poor old man from that home up the road". He was probably in a better position to buy drinks then anyone else in the room.

A woman of 84, mentally alert but paralysed down one side. She had no relatives, and friends who visited her told the Officer in Charge to spend all her money on her. She was financially very stable, clothes were bought for her and she was able to afford to go on any special outings etc. in fact she was short of nothing. A group of people visited the home from the community and the resident asked them to get her a nightdress on H.P., as she told the visitor she could not afford one. When the Officer in Charge heard about it, she waited until the group came again and called the visitor concerned into the office and asked her to speak to a Senior Member of Staff before getting residents anything and also told her that the resident had enough money to buy several dozen nightdresses. The visitor had said she had not taken any money from the old lady, as she had felt sorry for her. The Officer in Charge said to me "you know, Mr. Taylor this has implications out side the home and I am wondering what the visitor has said to her friends and if she has said anything, what will the story be like when they retell it". The same resident picked up her tripod and hit another resident with it. If she cannot get her own way, she will throw articles about and frequently swears at other residents and staff.

Staff, and new staff in particular, often quite unwittingly collude with residents in this sort of behaviour. For instance, a resident may ask a member of staff to make a purchase for them when they come back on duty. Many times payment is refused because the staff member feels that they are in a better financial position then the resident. Currently residents get £3.90 personal money. Those who smoke and take a drink are often subsidised by relatives. On the other hand those who do neither are quite well off financially, better then they have ever been before. They guard their money very closely and often hand over quite large sums to relatives when they visit, and need a great deal of persuasion to buy items of clothing which are necessary and will quite happily wear clothing acquired by the Officer in Charge, usually from a deceased resident or new ones provided by the Social Services. If a resident has been giving money to relatives and dies without leaving any for funeral expenses, the authority turns to the relatives and if they say they cannot afford it, then the authority must pay the funeral expenses and these relatives may have several hundred pounds over a period of time.

I have yet to meet a member of staff who is not of the opinion that the £10 Christmas bonus should be stopped for the old people in residential care, as they say it is usually given to relatives or goes straight into the bank and will eventually find its way to relatives on the death of the resident. I, personally, agree with this and am of the opinion that it should be divided up amongst the old people living in the community.

An old lady from a home went to the Dentists by taxi. The dentist asked why she should not have been brought by ambulance, as they were available to transport residents to the dentists. Enquiries were made and it was found that although ambulances were not provided for this purpose, the social services did provide transport for old people in homes. I wonder how much transport is provided for old people in the community, they have to make their own transport arrangements. I am prepared to gamble that many do not avail themselves of services they are entitled to because they cannot afford to pay for transport. Many authorities have holiday homes in various resorts and old people in Part 111 homes get subsidised holidays and, even then, many complain about having to pay and I know of residents who will refuse the offer because they think the authority should pay all cost. Old people in the community do get reduced rates for holidays out of season but even then the cost is far in excess of that for people in care.

I have already said it doesn't pay to make an effort on your own behalf and many old people who have had to go into Part 111 have found this out. Let me explain why. These are two couples, A and B. we will take couple A first. They have been prudent all their married life, worked and saved hard, bought a house, paid insurance to ensure that each would be alright should anything happen to the other and their children have been well cared for. Even in hard times they struggled on, as pride would not let them look for a 'hand out'. Always in the back of their mind is the thought that when they die their children will at least get the benefit of their efforts. Eventually, one of them dies and the other carries on until in the fullness of time they have to be taken into care – the house they own is valued and added to any pensions they have and also any money they may have in the bank. The old person may well find themselves paying full cost, currently in the region of £50 per week, though there is a sliding scale. The old person may live for a number of years in Part 111 and in consequence their assets will dwindle accordingly. Let me hasten to point out that they will not be put out when all their money has gone. When the old person dies and the funeral expenses etc. have been paid, the family get what is left which is often considerably less than their parents had hoped they would leave them. Couple B are the direct opposite to A. they have never saved a penny, never been inclined towards work or helping themselves, they spent all their money as fast as it came in. if they got into debt they would go to the Social Security, their children have been reared more or less at public expense. As with couple A, one dies and the other comes into care. They also are assessed and it is found they cannot afford to pay anymore than their pension from which they get £3.90 per week personal money and they will get exactly the same care as the remaining person from couple A. Some people reading this may think I am a snob wishing to segregate one group from another – far from it, as far I am concerned, if a person is in need of residential care then, provided we have a place for them, they should be given it. Let me develop things a little further. The two remaining people live in a home for a number of years and perhaps even become confused and unable to control their affairs. A bank account will very likely have already been opened for them by staff and, as they are not short of any material requirements, most of their personal money will be banked for them. Just for argument sake let us say £3.50. on one hand £3.50 is being put in and £50 is being drawn out. On the other hand the same amount is being put in and nothing is being drawn out. If both people are in care for a number of years, not an uncommon situation, one account is decreasing rapidly and the other is growing. I am not going in for mathematics but I think the message is quite clear. Over a period of three years B accrues several hundreds of pounds which, on death, revert to their family for no effort whatsoever and, on death A's family find themselves with a fraction of the original capital after all their parents effort and care. I question why in cases such as B the family should benefit from the efforts of others, namely the authority and staff of homes. I feel, and many residential staff agree with me, that in cases such as this, where money is accrued in this way after an old person has come into care, then it should revert to the administering authority on the death of the residents in part payment for the care they have received.

I relate the case of a lady who was in care for many years and did not smoke or drink. She resisted paying for any new clothes and would readily accept second hand ones. Her nearest living relative was a nephew who visited her rarely and then only after written requests by the Officer in Charge. When the old lady died she had £600 to her credit. The very day after her death, the nephew turned up at the home and asked point blank how much she had left. As her nearest relative he inherited the lot.

Taken for a ride – Michael Meacher

(66) Other instances of the failure to secure the anticipated or desired behaviour in various contexts from the confused also entailed considerable extra work for staff. Thus in the special homes residents known to be incontinent were regularly toileted once or twice each night, but some who omitted to utilize the opportunity promptly urinated within minutes of returning to bed. Again, residents who combined physical disability with mental confusion presented peculiar problems, like the obese woman of seventeen stone (confessional score 6), who either could not or would not get up out of her bath and had to be lifted out by force majeure by the matron's husband.

(69) Offensive eating, dress or toilet habits

Residents were asked, 'do you find any of them neglect their person, or because untidy, unclean or dirty in any way?' the replies indicated that feelings were most strongly aroused against incontinence, that little concern was shown about improprieties of dress, and that objections about eating habits, while sometimes appearing trivial, met with the distaste normally reserved even for small infringements of a strict code of conventions.

She seemed to be able to utilize' her confusion for the purpose of diplomatic evasion, sometimes with a faint ring of mocking derision.

Residential work with the Elderly – C. Paul Brearley

(67) Two particularly important aspects of physical change are incontinence and nutritional needs. Incontinence is important not only because of the distress it causes older people and those who care for them, but also because of the difficulties it creates in hospital and residential care and in transferring from the former to the latter. Incontinence can be defined as passed urine or faeces at unsuitable times or in unsuitable places (agate 1972). Most people who are incontinent can either be treated medically or can be encouraged and helped to manage their problems by habit training, improving accessibility of toilets, etc. some older

people are incontinent because of anxiety, depression or apathy; others regress and behave in a child like way, using incontinence to express aggression or hostility, or to further their dependence. The emotional element in incontinence can be an important one and treating the underlying unhappiness may help to build up self-respect and self-esteem and therefore encourage continence.

Residential Care Reviewed P.S.S.C. 1977

(91) It is important that incontinence in the elderly is not regarded by care staff as an irreversible process of old age. Its causes are complex. While medical condition can be the underlying cause, these can be exacerbated by psychological or emotional disturbance, or such disturbance may itself precipitate incontinence. Thus care staff should be aware that an elderly person may well experience incontinence for the first time on admission to a residential home and, moreover, that what might otherwise have been a transient episode can become a chronic condition by insensitive management. They should appreciate how deeply embarrassed most old people feel on experiencing this condition in the early stages, and should concentrate on encouraging such residents at every opportunity in re-establishing their pattern of continence. It should also be recognised that environmental factors may aid continence, e.g. the type of clothing worn by old person, the design and position of beds and chairs in providing easy access to WCs etc. the achievement of quick and unaided visits to the WC may well prevent the onset of incontinence, and may also represent a significant move towards greater independence and the maintenance of dignity.

When incontinence cannot be prevented, it should be understood that it is usually far less of a problem when all those involved treat residents as total human beings with awareness of both their physical and their emotional needs. Care staff should refer it to a practitioner since investigation of the cause may be necessary and there is likely to be involvement of the nursing team.

A wide range of aids for the management of continence is available (incontinence pads, urinary devices, protective garments with interliners, bed pans, urinals, commodes, etc). Social Services Departments should ensure that local authority and other residential care staff are kept advised of new items of equipment as they appear on the market so that the best choice can be made to meet the requirements of specially designed clothing available for use by people who are incontinent.

Do staff feel an over riding responsibility to see that residents are clean? If a resident is offensively unclean do they deal with it by leaving it to other residents to exert pressure, or by disgust, ridicule, persuasion or simple command? How much does it matter if a resident is slovenly or untidy?

Do staff know incontinence, the causes of it, and what can be done to help it? If not, is anything being done to teach them?

Chapter 13

It may come as a surprise to those people who indulge in 'Matron Bashing' that one of the tasks of an Officer in Charge is to protect residents from dubious friends and equally dubious relatives, particularly confused residents, as this group are the most vulnerable and are a very easy target for exploitation. Mentally alert residents have little or no patience with the confused and will shout at them, or just ignore them completely and, should the confused wander into someone else's room, they are likely to be met with a barrage of abuse. I know of Officers in Charge who have had rational demand that a confused one be moved out of the home.[70]

There was a resident in one home who never had a penny. She smoked like a furnace and spent all her money on cigarettes. The Officer in Charge began to think about the number of cigarettes she was smoking and how she could afford so many out of her personal money. A watch was kept on her and staff noticed she was always last to the dining room and first out. They soon discovered what she was up to. She knew who were confused and when they had been taken to the dining room she would take some money out of one or two handbags and then get back before anyone else and steal from a couple more. The residents she stole from were so confused they were quite happy if there were only a couple of coppers in their handbags and she was wily enough to realise this, so always left some cash to avoid the confused ones complaining they had no money. Staff took to collecting all the handbags at mealtimes or when the owner was not around to watch it. This particular resident then took to stealing from staff and was eventually caught red handed. The Officer in Charge had her in the office and warned her that if she persisted, he would put her out. He was bluffing and knew it but it worked. He said to me "We can't put them out, if she chose to she could steal other residents blind and why should others be exposed to this sort of thing"[92].

Many relatives and friends of the elderly are sincerely concerned about their welfare but there are also many whose visits are motivated by the amount of money they can get out of the old person. This group generate extreme anger and disgust in genuine staff of homes and in many cases, staff are powerless to do anything about it.

An old lady of 90 insisted on looking after her own money. Every time her son visited, staff found money missing from the handbags. He would tell her he was in debt and would be sent to prison. His mother gave him money each time, as he told her he could pay off his debts in instalments. Her family had only ever bought her two presents, both second hand cardigans and one was a mans. The resident became ill and the doctor said she was dying and, due to her illness, she became confused. Her son visited her. Prior to his visit staff knew she had £40 in her handbag and when her son left they checked her bag and found £5 in it. She was confined to her bed at the time she drew her allowance, £3.90, which gave her £8.90 in her bag. At this time, she took a turn for the worse and death was imminent. Her family were notified and it was agreed they could take turns in sitting with her. She died early in the morning. The relative who was sitting with her at the time told the Officer in Charge and left to inform the rest of the family. The Officer in Charge took a Care Assistant and went to the bedroom to perform the necessary duties and tidy up the old lady's effects ready for the family to collect. They checked the handbag and found all the money gone. One of the relatives had taken the £8.90.

There was a woman who had been in care for a number of years. She was a psychiatric case and had been confused for long time. Staff saw to it that she always had a few coppers in her bag to keep her happy and the rest of the money was banked regularly for her. She had a son who never once visited her. The Officer in Charge had written to him and spoken to him on the telephone a number of times requesting him to visit his mother but eventually gave up in disgust. When the old lady died, her son collected every penny which amounted to several hundred pounds and the Authority had provided everything for her.

A home took a "swap" from hospital. He was 80+, ambulant and quite continent, though deaf. The home were given no information about him so they set out to make their own enquiries. The found he had a stepdaughter and she was approached with a view to taking him but said she had no room for him. Staff said one strange thing about him was he ate like a squirrel. They then discovered he had a wife living in Warden Accommodation and the biggest surprise, the stepdaughter was the Warden. His wife took to visiting him and also taking what money he had. She bought him food which caused him to vomit. She was told he got regular meals and was asked to stop bringing food for him as it was making him sick. She ignored the request and the old man choked to death on this food. He had taken it away to eat it secretly.

It is surprising the number of people who, having got their aged relative into a home start telling staff what they should do for the old person. Should staff point out that there are 40 or more others in the home, they will be met with indignant threats of a complaint to the office or a Councillor. These people are often very arrogant and demand that staff of homes do what they, themselves, could not, or would not do. This is not peculiar to Part 111 homes. I have had it in Children's work and it goes on in all sections of residential care. Staff are aware that it is mainly due to guilt feeling and if a member of staff were to point this out to a relative, they would very soon find themselves on the 'carpet'. You can apply psychology for the benefit of your residents but it is considered very naughty to point out psychological shortcomings of relatives. They are the public- you are a public servant and servant you will be.

An old lady was admitted to a home and her daughter came to visit her. From the start it was obvious she was one of the type referred to above. Although there were no set visiting times in the home, the Officer in Charge did ask visitors not to come at meal times, mainly because visitors usually wanted to speak to senior staff about their particular resident and at such times, staff were always busy getting residents to and from the dining room and serving meals, so they were unable to stop and talk. Not so with this resident's daughter – she was going to come whenever she wanted and always wanted to speak to the Officer in Charge. It made no difference if the Officer in Charge was on or off duty, as far as the visitor was concerned the senior staff lived on the premises and should be available at anytime. Eventually, the Officer in Charge, a very patient woman, had had enough and the next time the visitor demanded to see her she invited her into the office and then very quietly and politely told her what she thought of her and her attitude, pointing out that residential staff were entitled to be left undisturbed during their time off. This resulted in a visit from a senior from the office. Even after explaining the problems the resident's daughter was causing, the Officer in Charge still found herself in the wrong and was told not to let it happen again but nothing was said to the visitor about being a little more co-operative. The officer in Charge took to being out whenever this visitor wanted to see her. As she remarked, "Being diplomatic is one thing but being completely servile is another thing altogether"[92] Some months after this, the resident became ill and was examined by the doctor visiting the home. He prescribed for her and she was given the medicine regularly but showed no improvement. The doctor and the Officer in Charge were very puzzled as it was not a serious illness and should have cleared up in a reasonably short time. As so often happens, the reason came to light by chance. The resident dropped her handbag, spilling the contents and a Care Assistant, helping her to pick the things up, found a container with tablets in it. The Care Assistant told the officer in charge what had happened and the tablets were given to the officer in charge who showed them to the doctor when he called. He asked to speak to the resident and asked her where she had got them from. It transpired she had told her daughter she was not too well and her daughter had gone to her own doctor and got a prescription (no-one knows what she told him), had it made up and brought it in without telling the staff. To quote the Officer in Charge, "the doctor hit the roof and his language was unprintable". He asked to see the resident's daughter and so the next time she came, it was arranged for her to see him at the home. He took her into the office and asked the Officer in Charge to be present. The Officer in Charge said to me, "Mr Taylor, that doctor had command of English which even made me squirm. He suggested to the daughter that if she wasn't satisfied with the care her mother was getting then she should take the old lady home and do the job herself and stop making life difficult for staff. When he finished with her, she could have walked through the eye of a needle". Things eased considerably for staff after this but the point is that the Doctor did what the Officer in Charge had tried to do and what her senior should have done months before.

Scapegoating is as common in Part111 homes as it is in other residential establishments but old people are not as resilient as children though equally, if not more, cruel to other residents. The point being that children are young and able enough to help themselves but many aged are not and cannot manage without assistance.

The new Officer in Charge took over a Part111 home where they were in the habit of serving tea from tea pots. The Officer in Charge considered this to be institutional (quite rightly) and announced her intention of providing small teapots for each table then residents would be able to help themselves and those who could not manage. The home had the usual compliment of arthritic, confused, blind etc. when the teapots were put out staff realised that only a few were drinking tea, the rest had empty cups. It was obvious that the able ones were making no attempt to help the others and the Officer in Charge suggested to them that they should. She was told point blank "No", they had no intention of waiting on others, that was what staff were there for. Even up to the time of writing, staff in this home go round at mealtimes and pour the tea for those who cannot do it for themselves. 71

In the same home, a borderline Educationally Sub Normal resident had her life made unbearable by another resident who alleged she had stolen 10p from her handbag. The Officer in Charge told me the home was chaotic for weeks and the E.S.N. resident was constantly in tears. The staff traced the 10p. the resident had spent it but refused to accept the fact and went on so long about it that other residents began to believe it had been stolen and sided with her. Eventually, the E.S.N. resident had to be moved to another home. 72

I have spoken to many staff about this sort of thing and the general opinion seems to be that residents will rarely help one another and sit around all day talking about one of their number, usually nasty, and seem to gain some delight in reducing the unfortunate one to tears. A resident who tries to avoid becoming involved by spending their time in their own room is regarded as a 'snob' or

(*E.S.N Educationally sub normal)

'too good for us'. Many staff says this also extends to day care as they are considered to be getting something the residents think they are paying for. One Officer in Charge said, "I swear, some of my residents would sooner see food thrown in the bin then given to the day care". 72

I have already commented on the attitude of the rational to the confused residents, so there is no point in going further with it but residents are jealous if they think someone is getting more attention then they are. I have spoken to staff who say if a resident is really ill and required a lot of attention, they generally get bitter remarks from many of the others because the sick resident is getting the attention. If one resident is taken ill, it is not unusual for several more to do so. Staff realise there is little or nothing wrong with most of them and accept it as one of the problems that goes with the job. Medication is another area for jealousy, the more tablets a resident has to take, t he better off they are – the status symbol.

Some even go to the point of refusing to allow one they dislike to use the lift with them and will endeavour to force the unfortunate one to use the stairs, no matter how incapable they are. It may surprise some people to learn that sometimes it develops into violence. I know of an Officer in Charge who had to break up a fight between two old men. I know this may sound funny to some people but I assure you, this incident was anything but funny. One man was very big and the other quite small and thin. Staff said, from what they could gather, the big man had been a bully all his life and to quote staff, "he's had his knife into the smaller man ever since he came here and has been continually goading him". Staff formed the opinion, after talking to the man's relations, that they were glad he was no longer with them because of his bullying ways. The Officer in Charge took the man aside and warned him if he did not mend his ways, a chair would be put in the corridor for him and he would not be allowed to sit in any of the lounges. The man started blustering and threatened to call the office and report the Officer in Charge. The telephone was handed to him but he declined to use it. The Officer in Charge then had some very hard words with him and made it quite plain that every resident in the home was under his protection and he intended to see they got it.

It is not unusual for residents to use their zimmers as offensive weapons. One old man hit a woman with his zimmer, knocking her down and breaking her arm. An old woman used her walking stick to trip anyone she disliked. There were several near misses due to this. Eventually, the walking stick was taken from her and she complained bitterly. It created extra work for the staff who had to assist her whenever she wanted to move but, as they said, there is less chance of anyone getting seriously hurt.

Staff of homes get bitterly annoyed when they accept a resident from hospital or community and find that information about behaviour or health has been kept from them. In the case mentioned above, the family know the old man was a bully but neglected to mention it until he was safely off their hands. The Field Worker was also aware of it but did not warn the Officer in Charge. All too often the residential workers are left to find out for themselves and this lack of communication can put them in a very vulnerable positions. 93

An old woman was admitted to a home for short stay, while her daughter was in hospital. When the staff helped her to unpack, they found a bottle of spirits and a bag of mints. The bed the woman was to occupy was in a dormitory type bedroom with ten beds. She was asked if she would like to have a bath. She said "yes" and in the process of bathing her, staff found she was covered in spots. The doctor was acquainted with this the next day and he examined her and prescribed. Over the next few days staff found she spent her time drinking spirits and eating mints. This also went on through the night. The floor around her bed was littered with empty sweet wrappers every morning. The Officer in Charge spoke to the doctor about this and he formed the opinion that the spots were probably due to this and advised the Officer in Charge to try to get the resident to stop drinking and eating mints, or at least drastically reduce it. This was mentioned to the residents and only served to antagonise her. By this time her daughter was out of hospital though still convalescing. The Officer in Charge acquainted her with the doctor's opinion and asked her to speak to her mother. She continued to supply the resident with spirits and mints. One night, the staff wanted to use some ointment which had been prescribed by the doctor on her spots. The old lady refused to allow them and they called the Officer in

Charge who took her into the bedroom and started talking to her about being so foolish. The resident threw her handbag the length of the bedroom and threw herself on the floor. The Officer in Charge thought at first she had slipped and picked her up. The resident threw herself on the floor again and fortunately for the Officer in Charge a care Assistant came into the bedroom just at that moment. The resident told the care Assistant that the Officer in Charge had hit her and knocked her down. The Care Assistant told her she was lying and that she had seen everything. When the resident left the bedroom she told the other residents and staff the same tale. No one saw fit to warn the Officer in Charge about the lady's temper tantrums or her continual drinking and eating sweets. The Officer in Charge said "Some residents are downright wicked. I've been in this work for fifteen years and that woman could easily have wrecked my career. The public would never believe how some old people behave and they will listen to them before us".

A confused old man was sent from one home to hospital and was discharged from hospital to another home. The only information the Officer in Charge was given was his name and the medicine he was receiving. The Officer in Charge telephoned the hospital and asked for his next of kin, age etc. two weeks went by and she had heard nothing so eventually, she contacted the first home. All they could tell her was his age, as all other information they had was passed to the hospital with him. When I spoke to the Officer in Charge of the second home she said the old man had been with them six months and only information she had was his name, age and current medicine. 93

There was a young man who ran a youth club. Every year at Christmas time he took a group of children to a home where they would hang decorations for the residents. He, in his way, was encouraging the children to be aware of, and show consideration for others. This particular time, the children had decorated the hall and quite happily went into the lounge to start there. They were met with abuse and driven out by the residents. The young man was told by them what had happened and he went into the lounge to speak to the residents. He too was abused and was told to get out and take his children with him. When he was leaving he said to the Officer in Charge, "I've been bringing children here for years and I never thought old people could be so cruel and wicked". They never went to the home again and it is staff who hang decorations now.

In conclusion, I would like to relate a comment by a Field Worker colleague. He was saying he would like to find some other work and at the end of our conversation he said to me, "You know, I think residential work must be the most frustrating job in the world".

Taken for a ride – Michael Meacher

(70) This alignment of the rational with the confused, with the consequent sense of unjustified deprivation among the former, was not, however, replicated in the other separatist homes. In these, greater implicit reliance was placed in the exercise of informal social controls by the reliance over their confused companions. In conjunction with evidence presented earlier in this chapter about the assignment of privileges this suggested a tentative typology of the distribution of power between confused and rational residents in separatist homes where by the more authoritarian the regime, the less the differential favouring of the rational terms of rights and opportunities and the greater their superfluous subjection to vicarious regulations.

(71) Assistance between residents

But if such excursions into real friendship across the boundaries of confusion were rare, did rational residents alternatively establish ephemeral links with their confused neighbours by the occasional service or act of physical assistance? Conversely, how far and in what ways did the confused offer such help to the rational or to others like themselves?

The support offered by the rational to confused residents seemed in both types of home to be of a somewhat random and unsystematic nature. In the separatist home, for example, a rational man from time to time offered a match and struck it for a pipe-smoking disoriented neighbour, who gratefully replied 'mark it up on the slate, even though the donor was well aware that his beneficiary never sucked hard enough to get the pipe alight and then requested help all over again. A hypomanic woman who was nevertheless ranked as rational on the criteria adopted here often led into meals a severely confused neighbour as well as two blind members of her dayroom; on another occasion, when a confused resident wanted a comb after a bath, she combed her hair for her, eliciting the remark that she reminded her beneficiary of her mother. A woman who was marginally confused in her speech and afflicted by a myxoedematous tardiness was meticulously attended to, not to say fussed over, by rational neighbours, one of whom would tie on her bib at mealtimes, whilst another would put her walking frame to one side and later return it to her, and a third would virtually combat the attendants against hurrying her up. Again a severely confused resident, whose behaviour was characterized chiefly by restlessness, disorientation and tangential speech, was assisted with dressing each morning by her placid rational bedroom companion, who also made the beds for both of them. Such instances as these are, of course, selective but they do illustrate the highly particularistic nature of such acts of assistance, their focus on the more moderately confused and their limitation to certain individuals.

(72) At the extreme was the habit of engaging in paranoid accusations: Mrs. Welson was notorious for her malicious slanders. Once on a coach trip, after quarrelling with the others, she shouted to the driver with animus 'they're all jailbirds – don't attend to them'. And when one of them remonstrated with her, she added, 'don't listen to her-she kicked a woman downstairs at the last home she was in'. On numerous occasions she called Mrs. Povie, her particular enemy, a thief and accused her and another of taking soap from her wardrobe. Mrs. Povie, coarse and aggressive though she herself appeared, was reduced to tears.

Residential Care Reviewed P.S.S.C. 1977

(92) It should never be assumed that the fact of residence in a home automatically restricts the rights and freedoms which those living in the outside community take for granted. By the same token residents are under an obligation to accept the rights of other residents, and of staff in the same way as people living together in a family. For certain reasons, some rights may have to be restricted, but such restrictions should be imposed only where individual circumstances leave no alternative. On these occasions reasons should be given wherever possible, to all concerned, especially to the residents and his family.

(93) If residential care staff are involved in pre-admission processes, the home will be better prepared for the new entrant. "if entry to this life was a gradual one the Matron of the home would have a true assessment of the said resident before entry, and this would also enable the Head of Home to receive Doctor's comments and case Histories before entry and not about one month (sometimes much longer) after admittance. It is very sad to see a person come into care and make an effort to settle in only to be told she is not quite suitable for this type of accommodation and that the reason for this is not what has been written into case histories, but more what has been left out!"

Such involvement also makes possible the early establishment of a working relationship between the home and the field worker. This practice should be encouraged. The field worker who knows the client and his/her background can be of great assistance to the residential staff in learning to understand him, and can provide a means of outside support for the resident once he is established in the home. The understanding gained by the social worker of the inside processes of residential care will also assist him greatly in helping future clients. Discussion should take place between home and field workers prior to the admission of a new entrant in order that plans for his future care can be drawn up and the responsibilities of both parties towards him be defined. Ideally the field social worker would be able to continue with his/her clients for an indefinite period after entry to care: however, we recognise the impracticability of this. But no social worker should close his/her file on a client before a first review has taken place and responsibility for the client should then pass to a specific residential social worker based outside the home, a resident should have this outside support available. Some authorities have a residential social worker attached to a group of homes for this purpose.

Chapter 14

I have spoken to many Officers in Charge about the frustrations they have to cope with and, without exception, they have questioned where "caring" is going at the present time as more and. more of their time is being taken up with staffing problems, work rotas, legislation, union agreements etc. These are all inter-related and if the present trend continues "caring" as many know it will very soon become an impossible task. I am not talking solely of residential care for the aged but all forms of residential care.

I have said "There is no one more alone than a residential worker with a crisis on his hands". Have you tried getting a senior to make a decision lately? When a residential worker asks for decision, they need it there and. then, not tomorrow or next week They are dealing with human beings and. are very conscious of the fact. I have seen Officers in Charge literally in tears with sheer frustration because no one would give them a decision and I have seen staff become ill with worry when situations have been allowed to drag on because those paid to make decisions consistently fail to do so, hoping if they wait long enough the problems will go. If the Officer in Charge takes matters into his/her own hands they may well find they are censured or reprimanded by the very people who should have done something in the first place. The fact that it may have been done in good faith and for the welfare of the residents is beside the point.[94]

It seems to me that caring for people is now part of the inter party, inter departmental, union/employer power game. One gets impression that "These care staff are a bit of a nuisance really but it does provide us with an excuse to set up the chess board".

You can ask for a decision from a senior or your union representative on any of the problems in this work and all you get is "it's a negotiated agreement, there's nothing I can do about it". With all due respect to employers and unions, this is not good enough. I accept there are bad employers but there are also bad union representatives and we are not dealing with machines. Negotiated agreements seem to have a definite industrial bas and shop floor tactics do not work in residential homes. We are not in a position to put residents into a state of suspended animation while groups sit around a table arguing. Residents are going to continue to function 24 hours a day and will need to be cared for because they cannot care for themselves. One might get the impression from the fore-going that I am anti-union but I assure you that I am not. I belong to a union and I believe sensible, responsible trade unionism can do a lot of good but I often wonder how much negotiators know about residential work. I have a friend in residential work who is also a member of the union executive and he admits quite frankly that when he goes to meetings and tries to put the case for residential work, it is like talking to a brick wall. He says other members see the world in terms of account books, machinery or bricks and mortar and seem to be incapable of thinking in terms of people who need to be cared for.[95]

Agreements may well be negotiated in good faith and yet nobody seems to bother getting these people together to monitor the agreements are working, and when agreements are abused negotiators seem to pretend the problem does not exist instead of getting together and confronting the guilty one and saying "That's far enough". Officers in Charge need some guidance on the interpretation of agreements and legislation -they need to know regularly what changes have been made - for the benefit of those responsible for policy making, it is called communication.

Employers have a statutory duty to provide an employee with a Contract of Employment. To me a contract implies a commitment by both parties yet this does not appear to be the case. Employers have six months (in the case of my own authority, 3 months) to assess whether or not an employee should be put on the permanent staff - the probation period. Now a foreman in a factory or on building site would probably be able to say in that time if the new employee was a good engineer, bricklayers etc. but I could not say in that time if a person would be a good residential worker even a field worker because of the intangibles in our work. There is no apprenticeship which can be served, when at the end of a given period a person becomes a fully fledged Journeyman a residential worker may only ever meet a particular problem once in the whole of their career. Residential workers with many years experience admit they are continually learning.[96]

Back to agreements;

People coming into the residential work need to have some commitment to the task, thankfully the majority of staff have but there are a minority who "play the system" and live on the backs of others. If a factory worker fails to turn in for work a machine can be shut down or the production line can be slowed but if a residential worker fails to turn up for work the situation does not change, we cannot put people into a corner and tell them not to function because of a staff shortage. Some staff will work overtime in an attempt to cover, many cannot because of family commitments, but mainly the burden falls on staff who live on the premises. Officers in Charge will often find themselves innocent pawns in a power struggle. They may have interviewed a person to work part time, say twenty hours a week on day duty. Initially, the candidate will be told that although they will be employed during the morning they may well be required to work afternoons subject to requirements in the home or the exigencies of the service. Upon agreeing to the terms the person will be engaged and it is then likely that for six months or more the new staff will work mornings only, then, due to sickness and shortage of staff, they will be asked to work afternoons until the situation returns to normal. The Officer in Charge will be met with the reply "I'm not doing afternoons, I only work mornings". If the Officer in Charge reminds the person of their agreement at the interview and insist it is honoured they are told "I'm going to the union". When the Union Rep. or Shop Steward is called in the Employer and the Officer in Charge will be told "By custom and practice, this person works morning and I am not prepared to agree to them working afternoons". Nobody seems to care about the problem of keeping homes manned other than the Officer in Charge and it is no use people reading this saying "Get more staff" - inexperienced staff however willing, can often be more of a hindrance than help, particularly when the home is short staffed, as there are none can be used to guide them.

I know of an Officer in Charge who worked 36 hours straight off because of all the situations I have written about. The particular home has 42 residents. The Senior Staff were the Officer in Charge, Deputy, Assistant and Senior Care Assistant. The Deputy went on holiday which had been booked for months, the Senior Care Assistant was off ill. Two days after the Deputy had gone, the assistant officer in charge went down with 'flu, five of the residents were in bed ill and three of them were terminal cases Two of the staff who were suspected of "playing the system" chose that time to go sick and sent medical certificates. One of them night staff and none of the day staff were prepared to do night turns and it was not feasible to engage temporary staff as it is necessary for night staff to have some experience. Whilst trying to sort out this problem the Officer in Charge realized she also had caught 'flu, yet as there was no one to fill the gaps she worked from 7 a.m. one morning through the night and all the next day. The doctor called to see the sick residents, took one look at the Officer in Charge and ordered her to bed. She protested that there was no one to direct the home. The doctor suggested a compromise. She would go to her flat and the remaining staff would. come to her for instructions. She had also asked a part time staff to change turns only to find herself in the situation mentioned above. I will not elaborate further on this case only to say that senior staff get the princely sum of £2.30 (now increased) on call allowance and they are not paid enhanced rates for overtime, very few complain about this but would like to see some justice. There are no 'perks', bonus schemes or productivity deals in this work.

Staff with a commitment to the residential task can justifiably feel bitter when they see others blatantly taking time off on the most feeble of excuses and then having to earn their money for them. A member of staff will openly boast it is easy get time off, just go to the doctor and tell him you have a backache or diarrhea as he has no way of proving otherwise you will get a medical certificate. The guilty one will then be seen perhaps carrying heavy shopping baskets or in a public house or one of several places and staff who have seen them will return to the home and ask the Officer in Charge why? Officers in charge become frustrated, helpless and downright annoyed when such situations occur. Manual grade staff are, because of agreements, entitled to full pay when they are off. If a rostered turn of duty is at weekend, then they are entitled to the full pay they would have received had they been at work or if a bank holiday falls into rostered time then they are also entitled to the day off in lieu. I know of homes where senior staff can predict when a member of the manual grade staff is going to be off. I quote the case of member of staff who presented a medical certificate just prior a Bank Holiday. As the rota had already been presented to all the staff and agreed by them there was nothing else for it but for senior staff to turn in and cover the duty. It was calculated that the staff put £30 in that person's pocket and this particular person was seen out on numerous occasions by other staff of the home and also got the bank holiday off in lieu.

I know a doctor who issued a medical certificate for two weeks and wrote on it 'headache'. Many doctors have taken to writing all sorts of absurd and silly words on medical certificates in the knowledge that the person was just "skiving off". It has occurred to me that they are trying to tell someone somewhere something and it is unjust and unreasonable to blame the doctor all the time if he /she is trying to tell the powers that be something, then it is up to those people to pick it up and do something about it. I also know of homes where a few of the staff go sick on a sort of unofficial rota basis - when one turns in another goes off. As have said, things do not change in a residential home when staff fail to turn up and I, like many others, think it is high time negotiators went back to the drawing board.[73]

I read a comment in one of the journals some months ago. It was about absenteeism and how it does not happen in residential work. I have no idea where this person got the information to make such a statement. I know an officer in charge who reckoned up hours lost for various reasons in his home over a period of six months and they amounted to *950*. Calculate that at approx. £1.12 per hour multiply it by the number of homes in an authority and it is a considerable sum. Is it any wonder residential work is considered to be expensive?

Another problem which is beginning to rear its ugly head is demarcation disputes. Although at present it may only be confined to odd members of staff, it is there and I have seen a growth of complaints due to this and unless negotiators on both sides of fence are prepared to learn something about residential work, results of their deliberations could prove disastrous for the caring function.

I know of a case where a domestic left a resident who had fallen on the floor and went to find a Care Assistant to help the resident up.

There is another case where a domestic refused to top up a bottle of detergent because a Care Assistant had used some when cleaning up after an incontinent resident. The domestic insisted that the Care Assistant refill the bottle before she started work

A Care Assistant refused to wash down some paintwork in the kitchen. She was not being asked to climb a ladder or stand on a chair, it was all below shoulder height and after some argument the Officer in Charge and her Deputy did it.

Where is this sort of attitude going to end? Who is going to look after resident's welfare if it is allowed to grow? I would to make one point quite clear to anyone who negotiates or has any dealings with residential work, everything involving work in a residential home is part of the caring function. In the last case above, the Care Assistant was asked if she would clean the paintwork in her own kitchen at home? When she answered "Yes" it was pointed out the principle was exactly the same. If the present trend continues, who is to cover the 'grey areas' residential staff?? If an incontinent resident soils himself/herself who should clean up the mess, the Care Assistant or a Domestic? If a resident needs assistance at meal times and the home is short of Care Assistants does he/she go hungry while someone stands on their negotiated rights and mops a floor. Alternatively, if there are no domestics on duty, should Care Assistants leave any mess until such time as they do come?

There are 'sea lawyers' in all walks of life, and residential care is no exception. From the time these types complete their probationary period dissention reigns. They will quote the union rule book, generate dissatisfaction amongst staff and will tell seniors what hours they want to work and also what hours others should work. The excuse is usually "I can't get along with him/ and (hand on heart) it is, "affecting the residents". The plain truth of the matter is that these kind of people don't give a hoot about the residents. They (the residents) are a convenient excuse to justify the trouble being caused. Unfortunately if such matters do get to the stage where the Union is called in, it becomes in turn another excuse for a minor power game to start again. If the Unions would only once in a while say to these people, "*You* signed on for this, if you don't like it, leave" but no, it is a case of who is going to win. The residents? Oh, yes, they are something vague in the background. I believe in a probationary period but if I had my way it would not be less than twelve months.

We now have the Health and Safety at work Act. Not before time in my opinion but it brings us back to the abysmal ignorance of the function of residential homes. In fairness, some Safety officers do use their common sense and do try to understand that staff are trying to create a home but there are those who can see no further than the Factories Act. As far as they are concerned if people work on the premises, it is a factory and the recommendations they submit make absolute nonsense of training courses for residential workers. This brings me to a problem which, if we apply the letter of the Health and Safety at Work Act, affects residential work greatly. In factories and places which would come under the meaning of the word, workers are supplied with equipment designed to safeguard them from injury and if there is any danger present, the employer/owner must inform the worker of its nature. Now, as I have said earlier, residential workers are open to verbal and physical abuse. Let us suppose a violent young or old person is admitted to a home and the person doing the admission or the family 'forget' to tell staff of the violent tendencies and the new resident attacks a staff member causing injury, where does the member stand under the Health and Safety at Work Act? I have asked several Safety Officers this same question and every one has side stepped it, yet these same Safety Officers check to see that all accidents are recorded and reported in order that they can conduct their investigations but they are conspicuous by their absence if a member of staff is attacked and injured. As I have already said there is a definite industrial bias to Union agreements/negotiations and whether we like it or not, that square peg is going into that round hole, if they have to use a steam hammer to do it. This also brings to mind Fire Regulations. It seems to me that no sooner does legislation go on the statute book than the left hand loses sight of the right hand. I have lost count of the number of times the Officers in Charge and private proprietors have expressed their concern at the recommendations made by fire officers. I was myself a fireman for a number of years and I am well aware of how great was the need for some tightening up of fire regulations but each fire officer seems to have different ideas about what is required and, again, about the function of residential homes.

There is the case of an adapted property with a ten bedded room on the ground floor where one fire officer said there should be a fire door. This entailed breaking through a very thick wall. It was done and the door was fitted with a panic bolt. A second fire officer visited and said a second fire door was needed. This also was done and again the door was fitted with a panic bolt. A third fire officer visited and said "Two fire doors are unnecessary, one would have been enough". This was not the end of it but I think the message is quite clear.

A new staff flat was built onto an existing children's home. Access to the flat which had it's own downstairs front door, was made through a gable end blank wall. The staff member occupying the flat asked if a lock could he fitted for security purposes as sleeping in would be done in the home and some of the children being what they are, she could see some of her belongings "going missing". The fire officer insisted that the door be marked as a fire exit and clear access to the stairs of the flat be maintained. He quoted the arguments and requirements of the fire regulations. The Home Officer pointed out that the flat was a private residence and the particular wall had been blank ever since the home was built, so why should a new door change things. The arguments bounced back and forth and I have no idea what the outcome was. I did suggest to the Homes Officer that the new doorway should be bricked up again and save all the nonsense.

Proprietors of private homes for the aged are concerned at many recommendations and often comply without question because of insurance.

One proprietor told me that the small print on his policy indicated that if the fire officers recommendations were not carried out his policy would be invalid.

Plain downright common sense is a commodity which is in very short supply these days and seems to get more scarce the higher one goes up the administrative ladder. If anyone in the Cabinet would like to create another minister, I suggest they make a post for minister of common sense.

I have made comment in this chapter on communication, or lack of it, as an example of the sort of communication we do not need, I recommend for your reading an article which appeared in the R.C.A. publication, 1978, Heads and Hearts. The article is entitled 'Communications between groups in residential care situations' by Robin Balbernie.

The article is spattered with the words, conceptualize – cogent - paradigm - ambience - oligarchic - coterminous and of all things concretize. I have looked in several dictionaries for the meaning of this word without success and none of my friends have been able to help. I can only guess he means something of solid mass.

I will not quote the whole article but there is one section which typifies the sort of gobbledegook which so many people in this work use to hide their lack of practical ability.

"There are similar happenings within groups. An affective boundary can be visualized as a semi-permeable membrane which passes (in either direction) units of information that are on average less emotionally charged than those contained within it.... (I have read this somewhere before! Residential work with Children - Richard Balbernie). This need not be coterminous with the official groupings, and can have 'intrusions' to seal off internal isolates 'extrusions' to include emotionally important others."

I must confess, I question the intelligence of the R.C.A. and Social Work Today for printing such an article and would pass on to them and Mr. Robin Balbernie a piece of advice given to me by a Psychologist friend - Communication is only complete when the recipient understands fully what the instigator is trying to convey.

Taken for a ride — Michael Meacher.

(73) Data already presented has demonstrated the staffing shortage, on a weighted basis, in the separatist homes, and at least in one such home exceptionally long, but fewer, shifts of twelve hours were opted for by married women staff, despite the likely decline in care standards caused by tiredness, because they offered longer unbroken periods of time-off. But apart from pressure of work and the effects of exhaustion, it may also be surmised that the comparative lack of rational observers in the special homes might undermine staff inhibitions against rougher or less sensitive handling of the confused at times of frustration because of their vague or slow reactions.

Certainly a number of incidents in the special homes, both related and personally observed, attest the force of these pressures.

Residential Care Reviewed P.3.8.0.1977

The Supporters

(94) The support may be provided by one person, or it may be better provided by a team, each member of which has particular responsibilities. It is important that the head of home can feel confident that decisions will be taken quickly or suggestions heard, and that her voice will not be lost in management before it reaches a level where action can be authorized;

Whoever gives the support must therefore have access to senior management.

The head and her/his staff also need someone with whom to discuss problems and who can establish a personal relationship with them. In this way they will feel a 'department' is looking after them, but that someone is available to them who is outside the main stream of line management and consequently less threatening, not a 'head office' figure. There are, however, disadvantages resulting from possible isolation from the department that may well outweigh the advantages. It can be useful for the person who provides support within line management to use the services of someone outside the management structure to perform some of his/her functions for him/her. Trained activity organisers or group work specialists do this in some areas. Teams providing support could draw in help from outside by co—opting people to work as part their team.

(95) Employers may be able to improve the efficiency of staff by providing support and counsel, and sometimes they can enable staff to realise their own limitations and unsuitability, encouraging them to seek other employment of their own accord. At other times, however, this may not be possible and in such cases it is necessary to face any publicity which may result from taking the case to an Industrial Tribunal. It can be helpful if appointments are made, in the first instance, on a six-month probationary basis with an option on either side to part before this period is up. This needs to be made clear at the time of acceptance since the pressure not to use this option can be very strong. Whoever has to make the final decision must be firmly supported, bearing in mind that staff duty is to resident and only secondarily to other staff, and that management have a duty to support them in this.

Information of all kinds should be passing continually from those providing support to the head of home and his/her staff. It is extremely useful if information can be gathered together in written form to provide a handbook for the head of home. It can include such matters as statutory requirements, legislation, centre's of advice and information on specific subjects, places where aids and equipment can be obtained, services such as occupational therapy and physiotherapy, medical facilities, training facilities and local amenities useful for residents. This can be produced in typewritten form and cost very little.

(96) All staff, including domestic staff, should be required to understand the basic principles of residential care, the specific objectives of the home in which they are working and their own role in relation to these objectives. It should be part of the responsibility of the head of home supported by management, to see that these are understood.

All staff, including domestic staff, should know and be able to explain, if called upon, the principles of residential care, the specific objectives of the home in which they work and their role in relation to these objectives.

Chapter 15

I recently read a short article in Social Work Today. It was regarding the quality of life for the elderly in care made by an eminent person in Age Concern. Among the suggestions made were participation in the running of the home, residents committees, representation on management bodies and choice in day to day life. There have been for some time, similar comments made by equally knowledgeable people, old people being responsible for their own drugs, collecting their own pensions, individuality etc.

Let me say here and now, that these people by their comments, display their ignorance of residential care for the elderly as it is today and I say to them "You are out of touch and 10/15 years out of date, and that this also applies to what is currently being taught on courses". May I expand on some of these suggestions?

One Officer in Charge I know well started a residents committee. All the members were elected by a properly organised vote. One resident elected had served on committees before coming into care and being something of a strong character he was able to manipulate the others and in some instances it was found he 'bullied' some of the others to vote his way. It soon became apparent that the home was being run to suit him, not the majority of residents. This caused a great deal of dissention and eventually the residents refused to have anything to do with it. I will not elaborate further except to say, if the majority of the residents are confused, anyone wishing to gain power in a home would find a very easy task and the democratic process would make life unhappy for quite a number.

An Officer in Charge decided to press for a bar in his home. The residents-committee were all in favour and promised to play their part in serving etc. All went well for the first few months then gradually the enthusiasm waned until eventually only one resident displayed any interest. I asked the Officer in Charge he would do when this resident finally gave up and he replied, "I will run it for them myself and I would advise anyone who undertakes this sort of thing to be prepared to do the same".

I can just see some of the residents we cater for at present collecting their own pensions. Most of the money would be given to the first person they met or thrown away and the Officer in Charge would have the devil's own job getting it from those who did return to the home with any or all of it. As for handling their own drugs, it is obvious that the knowledgeable have not seen what some residents do with their medicines and pills if they are not watched.

I can imagine the scene, "Don't you feel well love? I had that last week and I got some of these green pills. I felt a lot better after I started taking them. Here you try some? These red ones the doctor gate you aren't doing you much good". A confused resident wanders into another residents room and finds a bottle with coloured 'sweets' and eats them with possible disastrous results. Who is going to be held responsible? You will get no prizes for guessing correctly. Certainly not the people who advocate such practices.

There was an old lady in a home. Staff were told that prior coming into care she had tried to commit suicide. Over a long period of time everything was alright and no problems were experience. The resident, much like any other, would ask for something to relieve a headache and like others was given tablets which at the time were considered safe. One evening a member of staff noticed she had a small brown pill bottle in her hand. She refused to part with it and the Officer in Charge when called, forced the residents hand open, took the bottle and found four of the headache tablets. It was also discovered that she had more in her mouth, when the staff finally got the tablets from her mouth they counted eight She had been saving the tablets with the intention of taking them all at once. Had she succeeded she would most certainly have died.

Old people, if left to themselves with drugs, will swap them with other residents. Many, like children, consider the colour to be the important thing. I witnessed this in one home. The Officer in Charge was giving out the medicines after the evening meal and old lady demanded to be given a green pill just like another resident at the table. If staff fail to ensure that residents do take their pills it is not unusual for residents to go around choosing the one they want to take.

It is surprising the number of relatives and friends who take patent medicines and even prescriptions into homes unknown to staff. They make no enquiries whether or not the old person it is intended for is on a course of drugs already in spite of all the publicity regarding certain drugs reacting adversely on one another. The same people would not dream of doing this if the old person was in hospital for if they did the roof would lift. Some courses of drugs also require the recipient to be put on special diet. The old person only has to say to a visitor that staff are not feeding them and the very food the old person is not supposed to have is provided secretly and eaten the same way. Old people can become obsessed with bowel movement. They ask visitors to bring laxatives in for them. They not only take them themselves but will also distribute them to others. The next thing staff are faced with several cases of diarrhoea. The doctor is called and prescribes accordingly, the bowel movement slows down and the process is repeated. Even alcohol can be dangerous when taken in conjunction with some drugs yet people who are supposedly concerned about the welfare of a relative very rarely ask what is safe to bring in. The last thing staff of homes wish is to deny old people their favourite food or tipple. All they ask is the application of a little common sense.

Residential workers in all fields are concerned about their charges. They do worry about old people vegetating but how can anyone with any real knowledge of the work talk about individuality and then generalise?

If a resident -be they children, mentally handicapped, or aged, decide they do not want to engage in an activity, what are staff supposed to do? Put their arm up their back and say. "You will". As far as the elderly are concerned, the majority do not want to be bothered and make this quite plain. With children and mentally handicapped, there are limits to what can be reasonably expected from staff. The trouble is the knowledgeable seem to have unlimited access to the media or the propaganda machine and the very last people to be consulted are those doing the job. Residential staff are not expected to he human - they are expected to be superhuman.

There is the case of an old lady in a home which encompasses all I have said. She is deaf, blind, diabetic and doubly incontinent (Obviously a social problem!). She refuses to take any medicine until an imaginary doctor she talks to gives his permission. When staff want to give her medicine~ they have to shout at the tops their voices to this 'doctor'. If the resident cannot hear what they say she will not take her medicine.

Some visitors who have been into the home complained about staff always shouting at residents and how terrible it was etc.

I have not heard of many children jumping the queue for residential places but it is a different story with elderly or mentally handicapped. I know of one man in a Mentally Handicapped Hostel who goes home every weekend. He goes on Friday night alone and returns on Sunday evening. Staff say he is high grade and no trouble at all and are of the opinion that he could live at home and leave a place for someone far more in need. Approaches to the family over a number of years bring forth the same response, "We can't cope with him".

Old people are taken into care for a short stay at the request of relatives while they go on holiday. It is surprising how soon family conflicts develop. especially when they find that old person is clean, warm and well cared for and staff are told the family have no intention of having the old person back or the resident says they are always having trouble living with the family. It is equally surprising how quickly conflict is resolved when it is apparent that the old person will be staying. I know of a case where an old lady refused to leave and defied the authority to put her out. She is mentally alert and quite fit. She goes out regularly and treats the home like a three star hotel. The fact that there are dozens of old people in the community who desperately need to be in care does not bother her or her family.

I was talking to a member of a Social Services Committee and the conversation got around to Children in Care. I was trying to explain to him the problems staff have to cope with. He was obviously sceptical so I said, "How would you like it if some child called your wife an F...... old cow?" His comment was. "They don't really speak to staff like that do they'?" I told him I had only quoted a very very mild case.

May I offer another quotation? It is better to remain silent and be thought a fool than to speak and remove all doubt.

In a Children's home, staff often find themselves placed in impossible situations due to the type of child placed with them. Children (and they can be up to 18) who should be in a Remand home will be placed with staff who have neither the expertise or facilities to deal with them and these placements are usually by people who are too wooly minded to face reality. Many residential staff running family group homes do a fantastic job of providing a warm, caring environment for children who have been deprived of them and without appearing to be patronising or denegrating, they make good 'Mums and Dads'. They are not equipped either mentally or physically, to cope with young thugs. Many, many hours of work are given free for the welfare of their charges and it is this very willingness which is their own undoing because seniors, field workers and administrators abuse their devotion to caring for children. One very senior field worker received some very bitter complaints from residential counterparts about the type of children he was having placed in small family group homes. The field worker replied, "They will just have to get used to it. They are going to get more of this type". This was from a man who was heard to openly admit he had got out of residential work because he could not stand the pressure. I must confess the intelligence of such people, or lack of it, leaves me gasping. I admire these residential workers for the job they do and get bitterly annoyed when I hear of some of the placements they are forced to take.

I do not wish to convey the impression that residential workers are God's gift to Social Work. I have already said that dubious types gravitate to this work but when they are found condemnation, like the rain, falls on good and bad alike. I have reached the stage over the years that when I read or hear about residential worker being accused of malpractice, cruelty etc. I wonder to myself what caused it? What pressure has this person subjected to over how long? I have seen people behave in a manner completely out of character due to the continual stress impose upon them by an indifferent system. It tears people apart. I understand from various publications than an investigation committee is currently being set up to look into stress in residential work. I, like many in the work, will be interested see how the committee quantifies stress, also what type of people will form the committee. Will they take up post in various homes and work as an ordinary member of staff in order to gain first hand experience or will they just observe and speculate?.

With monotonous regularity, we are forced to suffer industrial action from various groups who claim special consideration. The reasons and excuses for demanding more money are legion, unsocial hours, dirt money, money for working in foul atmospheres and, latest, going to work when it is wet. If these people would really like to know what unsocial hours are I suggest they become residential workers. Forty hours a week is the exception rather than the rule. If you doubt me, just look at the time taken and tasks involved in running an ordinary home and, then if you can relate this to running a home for up to twenty children or thirty to forty mentally handicapped or old people with only yourself/one other on duty when half the residents may need assistance/ bath, undress or even move. How would they like to perform a manual bowel evacuation or deal with the smell from a colostomy bag or go out whatever the weather to get a prescription made up, often at very short notice. Then there are the bedclothes from incontinent residents or faeces on the floors and walls.

We are now faced with the paranoia of financial cuts and screams of horror at the amount of overtime in residential homes. The cuts are demonstrating one thing and that is this. What authorities are paying for now is what they have been getting free for years and I will tell these authorities now that the overtime which is being claimed by the majority of residential staff is not all that is being worked. Authorities are still getting a lot free time. The very people who complain set the tone. Like them, residential workers expect to be paid for working. They care for those whom relatives cannot or will not care for.

Are residential workers now going to be expected to step back several years and to work sixty or seventy hours per week for forty hours pay?

There is an old lady in care run by authority B. Her own authority A is 250 miles away and they pay B for her care. This lady has been in B's home for several years and whenever her own authority wanted to know how she was, they would telephone the Officer in Charge of the home. One day, the Officer in Charge received a telephone call from a senior social worker in authority A to say she was going to visit the resident. She duly arrived following day. It came out in conversation that her authority created the post as they believed in personal contact with clients and she had saved her authority money by coming on the train instead of using her car. She spent an hour with the resident and before leaving commented that the resident was having bowel trouble. Officer in Charge said he was well aware of it as they had to do a manual evacuation on occasions and also they had been caring for the old lady for a number of years and although she had been brought to them with no background information they had, over years, found out all they needed to know. The senior was asked if she intended returning to her own authority that evening. She said she was not and intended staying overnight. This lady travels around visiting people from her own authorities who are being cared for elsewhere. I reckon the cost of this one journey plus subsistence to be in the region of £50 or £60. The point I want to make is this. Authority A have been most vociferous and wringing their hands about having to cut hundreds of thousands of pounds off the Social Services budget, they have complained about having cut meals on wheels, home helps etc. and the hardship it will cause to the old in the community. I could tell them where to start cuts. Multiply £50 per week over a year and you can buy a lot of meals on wheels or home help.

Residential Care Reviewed P.5.5.0.1977

Residents' Meetings.

Regular meetings at which people can discuss in a relaxed manner all aspects of their life and work can resolve many tensions and avoid the need for formal complaints to be raised. Residents' meetings can perform a similar function to staff meetings.

Residents may fear retribution if they make complaints about staff; or feeling unwilling to complain because of a feeling of indebtedness; feel the complaint does not merit a formal procedure; or make a complaint about a trivial matter rather than point to an embarrassing but justifiable complaint. Similarly, staff may hesitate to complain formally out of fear of reprisals, or out of a sense of loyalty to other staff. For this reason it is necessary to provide an informal means of airing complaints. The arrangement of staff and residents' meetings has already been discussed.

Such meetings have their limitations as forums for complaint, but the chance to discuss freely and informally can be very helpful and defuse potentially explosive situations, as well as settling trivial matters. The greater opportunity of contact with people outside the home for both staff and residents, the greater the chance that complaints will be heard, discussed and dealt with by either informal or formal means.

Short term admissions

Admissions for short—term care are increasingly valued as a means giving relief to families caring for a relative, or of enabling a person remain in his own home for as long as possible by giving him temporary periods of residential care. This practice should be encouraged. The use of residential homes for this purpose can also enable those recovering from mental illness, or elderly hospital patients, to receive the kind of care and support necessary to aid their return from hospital to the community. The provision of short-stay beds allows too for flexibility.

Many residents hold their own pension books and handle their own money if they are able to do so? If not, is this because of administrative convenience? Is this considered more important than encouraging independence in the resident?

If there is fear of the resident being exploited or proving incapable, have the risks involved been discussed with higher authority and support been asked for if it is thought that there is value in taking them? Is the term 'pocket money' used, with its implication that this finance is a gratuity? Has any system been adopted for 'banking' residents money in the home? Is it explained to fee-paying residents that the quality of service is not dependent on the ability of the residents to contribute financially? Is it understood that false expectations may have been aroused in residents prior to entry?

Chapter 16

Mine is not the field of Mental Handicap though for the last few years I have had a fair amount of contact with residential workers with this group and as my own authority have only three mentally handicapped hostels and two workshops, I have again drawn on the experience of staff in other authorities. As it turned out it was to my advantage particularly for the purposes of my writing this book.

Whatever the faults are in my authority (and none are perfect) in comparison to others our mentally handicapped residents do very well. There are a lot of comments from related associations about the mentally handicapped being exploited. In some circumstances this is fair comment but it is unjust and unreasonable to generalise and, as the following pages will show, in this, as in other residential work administrators, councillors and pressure groups show a disturbing lack of knowledge.

Currently we see mentally handicapped workshops having the name changed to Social Training Centres (I would like you to keep this in mind as you read on). Not so long ago we were all treated to a campaign encouraging people to accept the fact that some people were handicapped mentally and society should recognise and accept the fact - fair enough, but is changing a name going to change the object of an establishment? Are the people who dreamed up this idea trying to hide the fact that there are mentally handicapped and that there are establishments which cater specifically for this group of people? What shall we call the hostels in future - Homes for the socially Inadequate, or Social Rehabilitation Hostels. The same thing happened over Approved Schools which you know are now Community Home Schools. To my knowledge the type of admission has not yet changed and I doubt very much if a change of name will have much effect on the mental ability of those who work in the establishment. As the great Bard said, "What's in a name?" Forgive me if I digress a little but for some years now I have seen euphemisms used more and more and I get the impression that those responsible seem to think that by changing a name the problem will diminish and hopefully go away. As in residential work, it is not the name of the establishment which matters but the quality of staff employed there and the willingness of administrators to make an effort to learn something about the objects of these establishments and in some cases accept their limitations.

A mentally handicapped man was admitted to a hostel. He was considered high grade and the consensus of opinion at the Case Conference was, that with a period of training and rehabilitation he would be able to manage in a flat of his own. A very senior officer in the department was involved in this case. The new resident was duly admitted and two months later the Senior Social Workers contacted the Officer in Charge and asked if the resident was ready for discharge. When he was told that a "period of rehabilitation" could mean twelve to eighteen months, or more, he was most annoyed. From his attitude the impression was formed that he thought a mentally handicapped hostel was a production line. IQ56 went in one end and in a few weeks IQ 100 came out the other.

I spoke to an Officer in Charge of a mentally handicapped hostel about the renaming of the mentally handicapped workshop. He produced for me six wage packets, five of which contained 5p. The Sixth contained 1p. Yes 1p. It appears that in this particular authority, residents have to pay for meals taken in the workshop £1.40 per week and, at the time of writing, several of the residents are in arrears to the authority to the tune of £11 and £16 because they are not earning enough in the workshops to cover the weekly cost. The Officer in Charge having been in dispute with the authority for years over this has now given up the battle. He said he refused to open the wage packets and gave the residents the money out of his own pocket. He maintains that the authority already have been paid by the D.H.S.S. the residents receive £19.50 from the D.H.S.S., they keep £3.90 and the rest goes to the authority for their board. This authority excuses the practice by saying it encourages the mentally handicapped to take more responsibility for their own welfare. The Officer in Charge remarked to me that he told his seniors he would not interfere in the resident's social education and if that was what it meant he wanted nothing to do with it.

To me, it is an affront to human dignity. The Officer in Charge receives continual reminders about the outstanding debts for meals but now refers the matter to the Social Training Centre? The cost of producing these wage packets and slips and the administrate requirements would be better given to the residents as pocket money. It would be interesting to ask if this particular authority are contemplating charging residents for meals taken in the hostel when the workshops are closed?

I went to visit one Officer in Charge and his desk was littered with the usual mass of papers and forms. I asked him how he felt about that sort of thing as apposed to being a residential social workers. He said, "I don't regard myself as a residential social worker, Mr Taylor, I consider myself a carer. I'm not a clerk, accountant, administrator etc. I deal with living beings". He became somewhat irate and went on, "I get people from the office coming here and carrying on because this form or that return hasn't been completed yet. They don't seem to care that there is a resident who has just shit himself and is trailing faeces through the hostel and I am short staffed, coupled with the fact that I have to be my own joiner, electrician etc., besides continually thinking up new ways of motivating and extending residents".

Where mental handicap is concerned, the High Grade know what a £1 note is and they also know what bonus is. The Low Grade can work just as hard in their own way as the High Grade and, if as in this particular authority, their work performance is judged against others then they can never hope to achieve any degree of success. Any sense of achievement developed in them by residential staff is effectively destroyed at the end of every week by the 'system' which prevails in the 'Social Training Centre' and is also compounded by sheer inexcusable ignorance of the administrators. I can only assume that these people see what to them is an adult but cannot see the mind of a small child and what is even worse, they made no effort to try and find out or understand. I asked an Officer in Charge if he had visits from any of his committee members. He said in the nineteen years he had been there he had only seen two, one of whom called in because she had lost her way and wanted some directions. The other was on an official visit during the day when there were no residents in the hostel. I was told the only thing she said was that she had noticed a broken light shade. The Officer in Charge said to me, "You know, Mr. Taylor, she missed the whole point of having a hostel, no mention was made of our function or what we were trying to do or the problems we face with this type of resident". He pointed out a resident who also had (Downes Syndrome). He said this particular resident was so severely handicapped that just to get him to put his coat on to go out to work was a major achievement. So far as the resident was concerned, he was going to work and that gave him some dignity the same status as the others but the poor chap was in debt to authority for his meals at the centre and getting deeper in debt every week.

In my own authority's workshops the mentally handicapped employees are judged on their own individual performance. Everything is taken into account for bonus purposes, Mental ability, behaviour, attitudes and effort. They all get a basic wage and the 'extras' are earned in one way or another and it is very rare for any one to finish the week without having something more than the basic wage and this is paid to the resident even if they are off ill or on holiday. There is a continuous assessment of the individual capabilities and as long as they work up to their potential, staff are satisfied. I understand from staff that the low grade tend to get more bonus as they are usually more amenable to direction. It is utterly stupid to reduce a person's earnings if their intelligence is so low that they don't know why. Our residential and workshop staff seem to have quite a good relationship – perhaps as one man put it, "We grew up together".

Instructors need as much background information as residential staff, after all they are dealing with the 'body' for a good part of the day and one tends to get overflow situations and aggression carried from the hostel to the workshop and vice versa. Both residential staff and instructors encourage residents to save out of their wages and they all have a Post Office Savings Account. They also seem to have quite a good social life with regular club nights, weekend sports and outings etc.

Back to residential work. I know an Officer in Charge who took five years to get three residents to go on holiday alone and as he said "This is due to the incentive we as residential workers generate in them. If I told an outsider this, they wouldn't believe me". He encouraged them to go down to the local Tour Operator and get some information on holidays in Britain and then encouraged them to do what was required themselves. They did the work and he guided them. They had a good holiday and were very pleased with themselves. He is now hoping that next year they will take the initiative and make the first move themselves. Though not a mentally handicapped worker myself, I can well imagine the thought, effort and patience that went into this.

We are continually told that the mentally handicapped should be given more freedom. This, like so many other comments about residential work, is a blanket statement and I would ask which mentally handicapped?

A group of mentally handicapped were taken on holiday. Staff decided to give one young woman 'freedom'. She went straight to a chemist, bought three packets of Bisodol and ate them like sweets. This culminated in violent vomiting and she was taken to hospital. A short while afterwards she had to have a sub total hysterectomy. Admittedly, she would have had to have the operation anyway but the doctor said that the strain of retching had accelerated it.

Sometime ago, the Association for Mentally Handicapped had brilliant idea to get the mentally handicapped out into the community. It was "Let's go cycling week". On the face of it, was a good idea but, like so many ideas which come down from the ivory towers, little thought was given to the possible consequences. One Officer in Charge I spoke to said that when he got a request for his residents to participate in this cycling week, he ignored it because of an incident which involved one of his residents a few months earlier. He related the following story to me.

A young man mentally handicapped and epileptic, decided he would cycle to the workshops and back every day and asked if he could buy a bicycle. The Officer in Charge being a forward looking man said 'Yes'. The resident paid

£80 for a bicycle and started cycling to and from work. The Officer in Charge was a bit apprehensive but thought he would give the resident a fair try. All went well for a few days then one day the resident came home with a bad cut on his forehead and a badly bruised face. When the Officer in Charge asked what had happened he was told the resident had fallen from his bicycle. The Officer in Charge said to me "It was then my conscience pricked me. It is alright to say we can't shield residents from all risks but it is criminal stupidity to put other people at risk in the process. I don't know if my resident had a 'petite mal' or just did something silly but either way, on a busy road it could cause an accident". He went on, "Suppose you or I were driving along with our family in the car and a mentally handicapped cyclist fell or swerved in front of you, your natural reaction would be to try and avoid him and this could involve you and other road users in a bad accident, also putting your life and the lives others at risk. You have no idea that the person in front of you cycling along is mentally handicapped and due to their mental capabilities, is liable to do something you would expect from small child". It is worth thinking about.

During my talks with staff working amongst this group, I had the same complaints about Field Workers dumping, (I have my own opinions on this but more of it later), lack of knowledge about the client and arriving at decisions without reference to the residential staff.

There was a young woman, not particularly mentally handicapped, who was placed in a hostel. After some weeks a case conference called, without the Officer in Charge's knowledge. It was decided she would stay in the hostel because if they let her go home she would kill her mother's baby. The Officer in Charge was acquainted with the decision which stunned him. He had not been at the case conference, no one had sought any information from him. and not one Field Worker had been to see him or the girl since she had been placed.

A young woman was placed in a Mentally Handicapped Hostel by a Senior Social Worker. Months went by and no one called or asked about the girl. One day, this particular Senior arrived at the home and asked how M.. and her baby were doing. The Officer in was very puzzled and asked what he meant. It was then the story came out. The Senior had met the young woman in town the previous week and when asking her how she was, he was told she had given birth to a baby and that she went to hospital every afternoon to feed it. He had assumed that the staff of the home were keeping it from him. The Officer in Charge told him that if he made some effort to keep in touch with them, he would be aware that she lived in a world of fantasy. The Officer in Charge said to me "I never go to the younger Social Workers for advice Mr. Taylor, if I want to know anything I go to someone who worked with this group back in the old welfare days". He did not say this with the intention of insulting Field Workers and after some discussion I discovered that his views on generic social work were very much the same as mine. I have spoken to a number of Field Workers and colleagues who agree with me that generic social work has caused more problems than it has solved. My own opinion is that a person, no matter how committed, cannot be all things to all people. When we had specialists in various fields, they not only knew the legislation relating to their particular group but they also built up a store of practical knowledge which was priceless. Today, a Field Worker is expected know the law relating to all the different client groups. This to me, is totally unreasonable. As so often happens in this work when the Seebohm Report was published it produced another syndrome, every authority had to go generic. I understand from friends it caused them more frustration than it is worth. Happily, some authorities have seen their mistake and are moving back to having specialist field workers. As things stand today, the emphasis seems to be on children and many people, both in and out of social work do not see the mentally handicapped, elderly etc, as coming under the social work umbrella.

Can I now go on to that argument provoking subject – Sex and the Mentally handicapped. I have discussed this subject with a number of people working amongst this group and so far I have found that those who are for it without reservation are usually those who have only worked with this group for a comparatively short time. Those who have been a long time in the work do have reservations and also agree that the mentally handicapped have physical and emotional needs just like any other person. One Officer in Charge had a

young woman with a mental age of 12. She went out one night and returned
in a very distressed state. He finally got the reason from her, she had been
seduced by a taxi driver. He said to me "You know, Mr. Taylor, that was a
traumatic experience for that girl. The only analogy one can draw is rape. I'm
not blaming the. taxi driver, all he could see was a buxom young lass who on
the face of it was willing. The girl is now afraid to go out". I would like to
say here that if a man seduced a normal girl of 12 he would find himself on a
criminal charge, because there is legislation the protection of young people,
but what is the criteria for this- mental age or physical development?

Another Officer in Charge told me he had two girls who, with the consent
of the doctor, were on the 'pill'. One was on it for menstrual reasons and
the other was promiscuous. He said the girls in the hostel were a constant
worry to him as none of them could cope with a pregnancy and also they
were very vulnerable and there is the added worry of V.D. He remarked, "If
a promiscuous girl caught veneral disease and passed it on to some of the
men, who then unknowingly passed it to some other women, what would my
position be then?"

Not for one moment would I wish people to get the impresion that I regard
this group as being different physically or emotionally to normal people, but
do gooders, pressure groups and other vociferous people who think they know
this work are very rarely, if ever, called to account when their ideas/demands
have been put into practice and raise a public outcry. If a Social Services
Department showed any resistance to ideas put forward by such people its staff
will be accused of being callous, indifferent, outdated etc., but when things go
wrong they remain strangely quiet. Explanations are then demanded from field
workers, residential staff and directors. More often than not it is the Officer
in Charge of the hostel whose head is 'on the block'. If I were the parent of a
mentally handicapped girl who became pregnant whilst in care, I would take a
very dim view of it, or even if it were my son who made a girl pregnant. [101]

I cannot see the Social Services Committee openly saying, "Go ahead, we
will take the responsibility", so who is going to? The people who are looking
after the body.

One Officer in Charge took a group of residents to a dance. One male resident had been taken to task on numerous occasions pestering female residents in the hostel. The Officer in Charge said the resident started making a nuisance of himself with some very young girls. He was warned about his behavior but continued to the point where it became embarrassing to everyone. Eventually, the Officer in Charge took him back to the hostel and told him in future such behaviour would not be tolerated. The resident had been taken out with the others on several occasions and each time the same thing happened. A member of staff who had worked in the hostel for twelve months thought the Officer in Charge was making a fuss about nothing and said so. The Officer in Charge told her if she was prepared to take full responsibility for the resident's behaviour, she could take him wherever she wished and gave her statement to sign to this effect. She signed the statement but took the resident out twice. The first time everything went well. But the second time they came back very late and she asked to withdraw her statement as she said she was unable to control him. The resident is no longer allowed to go to dances and each time he goes out he is accompanied by a member of staff. The Officer in Charge said, "He may be mentally handicapped but he is wise enough to know that if he bothers the older women they will slap his face so he goes after the little girls who don't know what to do when he starts his antics".

The following has nothing to do with sex but the underlying principal is the same?

The residents of a Hostel were taken to a local public house regularly. When they arrived the residents were allowed to drink in one lounge - two pints maximum. Staff sat in the next room so they could keep an eye on the residents and yet give them the impression they were managing alone. Some of the staff who thought they knew better complained about the residents being accompanied by staff and said they should be allowed to go and return alone and drink as much as they wanted. The Officer in Charge called them all together and tried to explain the dangers of such a course of action. He pointed out that it had taken years to build up a relationship and gain acceptance from people living on the estate. It was a tenuous relationship at best and if just one resident created a disturbance or was seen to be drunk, then years of work would be undone. His advice fell on deaf ears. He went on holiday for two weeks and staff took matters into their own hands. They allowed the residents to go alone and followed them down. Some of the residents became drunk and beyond control, several were sick in the hostel and were then banned from going out for a week. When they did go again they were accompanied by staff and took their drinks under close supervision. Staff were unable to repair the relationships with the local community before the Officer in Charge returned and, at the time of writing, he is still working at it. The Officer in Charge said, "You know, the mentally handicapped have a limit to their capabilities and it is time people recognised the fact".

Like other fields of residential care, staff that do not live in are, more often than not, never on the premises to face the consequences of any action or anything they have said earlier. This inevitably falls to the resident staff who will have absolutely no idea why a particular resident is upset or behaving in the way they are. Some people come into the work and are unable to develop the skill which marks a good residential worker.

I was in a hostel talking to the Officer in charge and it was getting quite late. A female member of staff was trying to get a severely handicapped resident (who I was told had not been well all day) to go to bed. The member of staff had been in this home for some years. The resident was resisting and I could see tempers on both sides were getting very short. The Officer in Charge made no move to interfere and I waited for the explosion. Just when thought it was about to come a young woman left the group and went to the resident and took his arm which the older woman seemed glad to relinquish. I was too far away to hear what was said but the resident calmed down immediately and allowed himself to be taken upstairs. The Officer in Charge said, "That girl is a gem Mr. Taylor. She is a born residential worker. As you saw she was obviously aware of all that was going on around her. She knew there was something happening which would have repercussions for hours and she stepped in at just the right time". I have already said that good residential workers develop a 'sixth sense'. Some pooh pooh the idea but it is true. I mentioned this to the Officer in Charge and he said, "You have just seen it in action". Without meaning to be disrespectful to the first member of staff I would say, as far as the work was concerned, her heart was in the right place but she was lacking that extra indefinable something which makes a good residential worker. The Second member of staff, although involved with a group was absorbing all the behavioural clues and subconsciously processing them, arriving at the right conclusions and course of action. Both were performing the same task with the same resident yet only one succeeded.

I recall a case I had related to me some time ago which I consider to be a piece of pure inspiration on the part of the staff concerned and epitomises the thought and skill which marks a good residential worker.

There was a severely handicapped man in a hostel. He was obsessed with the police and fire brigade. His room was full of toy police cars and fire appliances. Every time he went out he made his way down to the local Police Station -in fact he became something of a nuisance and, sad to say, some of the policemen used him as a source of amusement. The Officer in Charge was concerned about it all and went down to the Police Station and suggested to the Sergeant that they could help him, themselves, and the resident if they gave him something very simple to do like collecting car numbers. The Sergeant proved to be very understanding and agreed to help, so the next time the resident turned up he was told he was to be taken on the Force part time and asked to go to a certain part of the town, where there was a bench to sit on and collect the numbers of all the cars which passed. The resident was quite happy doing this and the station staff got peace. As often happens, one 'bright' person at the station thought they would have some fun at the resident's expense and presented him with a toy paper mache police helmet. This may have provided amusement for the station staff but it certainly caused a great deal of worry and concern for the Officer ,of the Hostel as the resident refused to part with the toy helmet and wore it every time he went out. This marked him in the community as mentally deficient and because of this, he was becoming the butt of jokes and cruel comments particularly when he was collecting car numbers. As the weeks went by, the staff became very concerned as the resident steadfastly refused to part with his helmet and could not understand he was making a fool of himself, after all, hadn't the police given him a job? The Officer in Charge's wife had a brilliant idea. She went to see the Inspector and told him about the problem and the staff's concern. She suggested that the resident be transferred or promoted to the Plain clothes Branch The Inspector proved to be very understanding and the next time the resident arrived at the Police Station complete with helmet he was called into the office and was told he was being promoted and would no longer be required to wear 'uniform' and his helmet was to be handed in. The resident, in his own way, was thrilled with his promotion and happily handed over the helmet and went out to collect his car numbers.

It is due to the above type of skill I get very angry when so called 'professionals' brush aside the comments of residential workers.

A mentally handicapped woman in a Hostel was thought to have dangerous violent tendencies. Staff had voiced their fears to the visiting psychiatrist on a number of occasions but he told them they were imagining things and he could see no cause for alarm. This went on for several more weeks with staff using all their skill to contain the situation. One evening when the psychiatrist was upstairs with another resident the woman burst into the office with a knife in her hand and started to threaten one of the two staff who were on duty. The second member of staff went upstairs for the psychiatrist while the first staff kept the woman's attention by talking to her. The psychiatrist walked into the officer and the woman turned and attacked him with the knife. The two staff had to overpower her and take the knife away - within a few hours the woman was in a secure psychiatric unit. I understand that after the incident the psychiatrist paid a great deal of attention to what the staff had to say about the residents.

One Officer in Charge I spoke to said he often wondered if severely mentally handicapped people could feel pain. He said there was a young woman resident in the hostel who had one leg shorter than the other. One day the resident was having a shower (a member of staff was present) and fell, knocking her elbow. She was assisted up and asked if she was alright. She said she was and next day, I quote the Officer in Charge; her arm was like a balloon. She was taken to the hospital where the arm was X rayed and she was found to have a bad fracture. The Officer in Charge said, "Most people would have been screaming with pain all night, but the resident hadn't murmured and slept well". He said he had heard of similar incidents but this was the only one he had actually experienced

Residential Care Reviewed P.S.S.C. 1977

Mentally handicapped people of all ages need a permanent home with a door wide open to the outside world for anyone who can become sufficiently independent to leave. The assumption should always be made that all residents will one day manage to do so, because behavior will frequently develop in response to that expectation.even if his development is not sufficient for the resident to be able to leave home, he will benefit from such an approach. In this sense a home for the mentally handicapped should resemble far more the 'family home' where the family members will always belong but from which they are likely to move out. It is worth noting here the danger of continuing to treat adult mentally handicapped people as if they were still children. This can happen more often in those homes which provide for both mentally handicapped children and adults, the children staying on as they grow into adulthood. Mentally handicapped adults need adult treatment: it is something which the parents of mentally handicapped people may find hard to give and which homes should be alert to provide. There is particular value in the provision of accommodation in which mentally handicapped people can try to live independently within the shelter of the home. Their right to a sexual life needs to be understood and accepted and considerable thought needs to be given to 'opening out' and overcoming the problems involved. Until this right is openly accepted, the necessary discussion of these problems, the search for solutions and provision of advice for staff are unlikely to materialise. Homes for the mentally handicapped come under great pressure particularly from parents and it is especially important that their objectives should be stated.

(101) Do staff feel that residents should not be allowed to form intimate

relationships or be allowed sexual freedom? If so, why? Is it because it often embarrasses the staff? Or because it offends the moral code of the staff? Or because they feel it might offend other residents? Do they believe they have a right to impose their morality on the residents? Do they believe it is wrong to leave it to the group to establish its own attitudes? Do they understand that handicap of any form does not necessarily diminish the need for sexual relationships? Do they realise how they can, both by their attitudes and also by practical help, relieve tensions and promote considerable happiness? Have they been given any guidance or help in learning about this?

Chapter 17

I t is now the 10th August 2005, and I am in my 78th year. The manuscript for this book was borne out of anger, an anger which was generated by seeing the way, staff of Homes for the Elderly were treated by those who ordered our lives, both national and local, and their woolly minded policy regarding young law breakers (Delinquents).

A couple of weeks ago, I watched a programme on the T.V. It was Panorama – BBC and was about how Elderly Patients were being treated in Hospitals, there was a telephone number at the end, for anyone who wanted to comment. I rang the number and asked the lady who answered, if the Hospitals were still bartering patients with the Residential Homes. She said, she didn't understand me, I told her what my work had been, and what I had seen. She said she would pass the information on to the programme Producers, and took my telephone number, she said, if they wanted to know any more they would contact me. I have heard nothing.

The Government are forcing Residential Homes to close pleading shortage of money, yet they can afford to build new Prisons. Also they can afford to give billions of pounds a year to a corrupt – wasteful – bureaucratic – monolithic organisation called the European Union, and another similar, but bigger organisation called the United Nations.

During my time in Residential Work, Politicians were warned, that to close Part III Homes, and leave the Elderly to be attended to in their own homes would not be cheaper, and with a growing number of Elderly, who would need care, it would be more expensive, this has now proved to be the case. It has also made the Elderly more vulnerable as news items attest.

A similar situation applied with Approved Schools, virtually all sanctions for bad behaviour were withdrawn. The results of this liberal thinking are now only too apparent, those who order our lives refuse to admit that it is not working, and never has worked. When children of twelve, and young people in their teens, are actively involved in murder and other major crimes then there is a need for desperate measures. I am very much in favour of Human Rights, but this should not be used as a shield of convenience. I am not in favour of brutalizing children, but they should be made to understand that 'Rights' have to be earned, and this applies to adult criminals. Anyone who abuses those 'Rights' should forfeit them, until such time as they have earned them again.

The Government is now proposing to pay young criminals to behave – to stay at school, and not to truant. Is this the modern version of 'Dane Geld'? That didn't pay either. Politicians continually tell us that the crime rate is falling. Do they really think that all the people are as mentally feeble as they are?

Years ago when Harold Wilson took Capital Punishment off the Political Agenda, everyone was talking about it, - was it good or bad? I happened to go into a works canteen, there was one man sitting alone, when things quietened down, he said it is a Criminals Charter. The argument started again, this man took off his shirt and turned to show his back, it was like a Railway junction, he had been flogged at some time, silence descended, he just said "I have never gone back for another dose, and I have not broken the law since."

People like me were "shouting into the wind", when we tried to tell those who ordered our lives. We were only the people who were doing the job, they were the ones who told us what to do, even though they had no idea what the work entailed, crime has rocketed over the years.

In those days we had heard of the Mafia, but we had never heard of the Triads or the Yardies, we have now, major organised criminal rings. The question has to be asked, "How were these major criminal organisations, allowed to establish themselves, and grow in this country?"

Ronnie Biggs was involved in a train robbery, which caused the death of a man. He escaped to Brazil with his share of the loot, and laughed at British attempts to extradite him. He married an Brazilian woman, he could then claim their Citizenship, this was fine for him for years. Then he needed medical attention, which he couldn't afford in Brazil, but he could claim to be a British

Citizen, and be entitled to medical care. Of course when he landed he was arrested and sent to prison, but he also got first class medical attention. When people objected, his son who came with him pleaded he was an old man, so he is, but not for him is the waiting to see a Doctor, not for him and his kind is the lying on a trolley for hours in a Hospital corridor, not for him the worry if their pensions will stretch for something a bit special in the food line, nor for them the worry of keeping warm in the winter, not for them the worry of Council Tax, when they go up and Pensions remain static, not for them the having to pay for private medical service ie surgery. They will not have to face being put to bed at 4.00 pm and being left until 10.00 am the next day, new Prisons take priority.

On the TV news today, one item was that one Prison Authority had spent £60,000 on entertainment for Prison inmates.

Young people who avoid Anti Social behaviour get no credit, young Delinquents get an army of people running after them, millions of pounds is being spent on them, if they are expelled from school they get one-to-one education. The Political solution to this is to throw money at it, when all that is needed is, a strong determined person with the courage to make them pay for every wrong they do.

The Mother of a lady I know was taken to hospital, she was in her 80's. She complained about having to lie on her back all the time, she said it was hurting, and could she have another pillow so she could sit up. She was told she couldn't have one as there was a shortage of pillows!! Her Husband went to see her, and found she was dead. She had died an hour earlier, but no one had seen fit to inform him.

Human Rights – Hooray!! Can anyone tell me where I can find them.

ISBN 1425103731

9 781425 103736